Nurses' Aids Series

PSYCHOLOGY FOR NURSES

NURSES' AIDS SERIES

NURSES' AIDS SERIES

PSYCHOLOGY FOR NURSES

FOURTH EDITION

A. Altschul

B.A. (Lond.), M.SC. (Edin.), S.R.N., R.M.N., R.N.T.

Senior Lecturer, Department of Nursing Studies, University of Edinburgh;
Formerly Principal Tutor, the Bethlem Royal Hospital and the
Maudsley Hospital, London; Formerly Examiner to the General Nursing
Council for England and Wales

WITH A FOREWORD BY

A. G. Caws

B.SC., Ph.D. (Lond.), F.B.P.S.

Formerly Principal Lecturer in Psychology, Battersea College of Technology;
Examiner for the Sister Tutor's Diploma, University of London

BAILLIÈRE TINDALL · LONDON

BAILLIÈRE TINDALL
7 & 8 Henrietta Street, London WC2E 8QE

Cassell & Collier Macmillan Publishers Ltd, London
35 Red Lion Square, London WC1R 4SG
Sydney, Auckland, Toronto, Johannesburg

The Macmillan Publishing Company Inc.
New York

First published 1951 as
Aids to Psychology for Nurses
by Norah Mackenzie
Third edition 1969
Fourth edition 1975

ISBN 0 7020 0554 1 Limp
ISBN 0 7020 0555 X Cased

Published in the United States of America by
The Williams and Wilkins Company, Baltimore

Printed Offset Litho in Great Britain
by Cox & Wyman Ltd,
London, Fakenham and Reading

FOREWORD

All nurses will find this book both interesting and challenging, for, while technical advances in medicine tend to encourage the view that the patient is merely a complicated anatomical structure, he is, and must always be, a living person with family responsibilities, personal worries, hopes and fears.

Miss Altschul, therefore, asks her readers to study their patients carefully and furthermore demands that they should study themselves, because one of the great truths in nursing is that the patient is affected not only by what is done for him, but by what is said to him and indeed by how those tending him feel about him. On reading her manuscript I was tempted to suggest an alternative title—'The Patient in the Bed by the Door'—but a descriptive title of this nature would belie the fact that this is a textbook giving details of scientific facts, experiments, conclusions and theories—a book as important and useful as any other in the nurse's reading list.

This book is concerned with ordinary people living their daily lives; there is therefore a danger that the ready acceptance of the general theme may cause the factual importance of specific topics to be overlooked. However, everyday happenings are often worthy of critical examination. What, for instance, is the effect of the phrase, 'He's getting on as well as can be expected', upon a household awaiting news of a loved one in hospital?

I was once told that a psychologist's laboratory is the street, the home or the factory. This, of course, is an over-simplification, for even observation of people working on a ward demands training in observation itself. In fact, many psychological researches have required the use of extremely delicate apparatus; but because the subjects of many of our psychological investigations are just ordinary people the student of psychology is given an opportunity not possible in other sciences. He can say, 'Are these facts in accordance with my experience?' 'What is the situation on my ward?' The conclusions drawn from such questions are not in the least likely to be reliable, but the importance of such queries is that a valuable attitude of mind has been set up.

This book, therefore, demands more of the reader than mere study; it suggests that nurses should discuss its arguments with their fellows and above all that they should read as widely as possible. Some nurses may be puzzled to discover that there appears to exist a divergence of views among psychologists concerning the theoretical conclusions to be drawn from their experimental data. There are indeed many 'schools' of psychology, for experimental psychology is a young science and has attracted many workers who received their basic training in other sciences. Psychology moreover is a 'bridge' science linking the seemingly exact sciences such as biology and chemistry with those which appear less amenable to statistical measurement—sociology for example. But because psychology deals with human beings in all their activities this bridge should also link the traditional sciences with immensely important topics involving philosophy and the fundamental questions of religion. All these studies have sooner or later to face the problem of the possible relationship existing between mind and body.

Some workers save themselves all thought by either denying any relationship or by stating that such questions should be the business of philosophers and not hard-working nurses. Where this is so Mr Jones in the bed by the door becomes just a diseased appendix.

Other workers do seek to find a relationship between Mr Jones's mind and his body. They, however, state that his mind is one of the results of his evolution from a much simpler organism. To them Man is indeed a complicated mechanism, wonderful in its intricacies, but nevertheless a mere machine controlled partly by its structure and partly by the circumstances of its environment.

There are other workers in the field of psychology who do regard Mr Jones as a unique personality whose mind is worthy of our most detailed study. Many investigations into the nature of the unconscious activity of the mind have been carried out and stress is rightly placed upon the need to recognise that many of our motives originate in such unconscious activity. Sometimes, however, the writings of workers in this field of psychology appear to give the nurse little help with her patient; indeed, the mind appears as a veritable bear-garden of warring factions. In this connection I have been much encouraged by the words of the late Professor Jung who stated that ability to recognise consciously the dark side and the evil within us is not enough. . . . 'Man has not yet been able single handed to hold his own against the powers of darkness, that is of the Unconscious. Many have stood always in need of that spiritual help which each individual's own religion holds out to him.' The importance of this spiritual factor cannot be overstressed. Some patients derive much strength from their religion because this can give the three great therapies of comfort, hope and courage. The spirit within the man is truly a force to be reckoned with when sickness comes to him.

All schools of psychology therefore can put forward only tentative explanations of human behaviour. This is why psychology is so exciting. Progress is very rapid in many branches of it, but all workers are finding the need to co-operate with the other biological sciences. The important fact to remember is that this progress should prove of real value in the lives of every one of us.

And what of Mr Jones in his corner bed? I would say to every nurse—Does the patient feel reasonably secure both with yourself as his nurse and with his fellow patients? Whatever status you may have in the hospital you have some control over both these factors. Furthermore, is he among friends? (I may feel perfectly secure in a crowded railway carriage but I am not necessarily among friends.) Do you respect him as a person in spite of his foibles? Has he, with due regard to his physical or mental condition, much opportunity to help himself? All such questions are good psychology and Miss Altschul will help you to answer them.

A. G. CAWS

PREFACE TO THE FOURTH EDITION

In introducing this edition I again draw the reader's attention to two points. The first is that both this preface and Dr Caws' foreword are intrinsic parts of the book and should be read with care. Dr Caws' foreword is especially valuable for it explains how psychology (and therefore my book) is concerned not so much with abstract ideas and theories as with 'ordinary people living their daily lives'.

Secondly, psychological knowledge forms the basis of good nursing, for nobody can nurse well who does not have some understanding of the psychological working of the human personality. To no-one is it more important than to a nurse that she should understand how people react to their upbringing, their environment, their health or sickness and their social contacts. The study of psychology is therefore an essential and most interesting part of the nurse's training, for, from such study, she learns how she herself and all whom she meets in hospital, doctors, nurses, patients, patients' relatives and many others react to the changing circumstances of life.

During the last few years psychology has advanced on many fronts. In nursing, this has chiefly served to furnish new practical examples and has helped to put the applications of psychological theory on an even firmer footing. No fundamentally new theories have clamoured for inclusion in this text. It is gratifying that an increasing number of nurses have found their way into research and that many of these make use of their psychological knowledge in planning their projects and test psychological theory in the nursing setting. Some of their findings are referred to in this edition.

Otherwise this edition only deviates from earlier ones in that most chapters have been brought up to date to incorporate recent writings and recent research.

I have divided my book into three parts, 'Psychology and the Patient', 'Psychology and the Nurse', and 'Psychology and the Hospital'. This division is not intended to suggest that each part is a compact and watertight compartment; on the contrary, 'Psychology and the Patient' contains much information that is applicable to the nurse's own personality;

'Psychology and the Nurse' contains much information equally applicable to the patient; while 'Psychology and the Hospital' should be understood to be applicable to communities other than the hospital. The book is a coherent whole and its division into parts is no more than a convenient method of arrangement.

It is my hope that every nurse who reads my book will find in it not merely the information she needs to help her pass her examination but, more importantly, a body of knowledge which will be a standby to her throughout her life. If, in addition, I succeed in so catching her interest that she discovers for herself the continued enjoyment to be gained from further reading and from more extensive study of the subject I shall feel well rewarded for the work entailed in the preparation of this book. Like other basic subjects psychology is usually taught early in the nurse's training. This book is, however, intended to be used throughout training because practical nursing experience will help the student to understand it more clearly and to collect from her own experience examples to illustrate the text.

I am grateful to my colleagues and students, past and present, for comments and criticisms and for the stimulation of discussions with them. Only some of these have been incorporated in this edition, others will provide ideas for more extensive revision at a future date. I should like to thank Miss Daphne Kennedy-Fraser, MA, ALA, for her valuable assistance in proof reading.

To Dr Caws I am deeply indebted for the help and support he has been giving me since the first edition of the book was contemplated, and for again providing the foreword to the book.

A. ALTSCHUL

Edinburgh,
1975

CONTENTS

PART III

Psychology and the Hospital

DEFINITIONS AND SCOPE OF
THE SUBJECT

Psychology may be defined as scientific study of behaviour and experience. This is only one of the many attempts to define a relatively new subject. Many people use the word 'psychology' quite loosely. They believe that they are using psychology in their efforts to cope with difficult people, in their skill in understanding others and in their method of getting their own way. Most people believe themselves expert in the art of living and of coping with their fellow men and therefore believe that they are, in fact, psychologists of a sort. Only when they find themselves in difficulty, when they feel mis-understood, or when it is evident that ordinary methods of approach are unsuccessful in dealing with others, do people become aware of a need for more or better psychology.

It is the purpose of this book first, to show what psychology really is about and second, to see if nurses, in any part of their work, can benefit from a knowledge of psychological facts.

Nurses, however well read in psychology and however thoughtful about themselves or other people, are not psychologists. A psychologist is a scientist. He or she has obtained a university degree in psychology and spends his working life either carrying out scientific research, thus adding to the body of psychological knowledge, or applying his special scientific knowledge to the investigation and solu-tion of practical problems in various fields.

In education, for instance, among much other investigation, psychologists have carried out research into the advantages and disadvantages of giving intelligence tests to school children, into problems arising when children are grouped in school according to intelligence or when children of all intelligence levels work together. Psychologists have studied children with special reading difficulties and have tested various ways of overcoming these. They have studied the effect of reward or punishment on learning. Work done with animals and human beings has helped them discover how learning takes place and though one can not directly apply findings from animal experimentation, subsequent research with human beings can advance understanding of children's problems.

The findings of the psychologists are available to teachers, who may or may not make use of them, but perhaps become better teachers when they do. However fervently a teacher takes psychological theory into account he does not become a psychologist, but merely a better-informed teacher.

Throughout this book there will be examples of psychological research and summaries of psychological findings which may or may not help nurses to become better nurses. Perusal of this book cannot and is not intended to turn nurses into psychologists.

Psychology is a SCIENTIFIC Study

Sciences are distinguished from other studies by the methods employed, not by the nature of the subject matter, nor the degree of certainty with which knowledge is held to be true. In physics, for example, one of the oldest sciences, or in chemistry, many facts which appeared to be definite have recently been disproved. Nevertheless, physics and chemistry remain sciences though truths are no longer proclaimed with the same dogmatic certainty as formerly.

Scientific methods consist largely of controlled observation and experiment. Casual observation of striking episodes or events often gives rise to scientific study, but in itself it is misleading rather than helpful. For instance, Sir Cyril Burt observed that many young offenders were of low intelligence. Though Sir Cyril Burt did not himself suggest it this observation was first held by many people to indicate a causal relationship between low intelligence and delinquency. Careful scientific research, however, indicated by his observation, has shown that this is not so. At the same time psychologists have become interested in much more important aspects of juvenile delinquency and have provided many useful data on this problem.

It has been observed that some children on leaving hospital have returned to bedwetting or have had nightmares. Some mothers have observed that their children are more clinging than before their entry to hospital. These casual observations are useful in that they point to the need for scientific research into the effect of hospitalisation on young children. Psychological findings are now available and nurses are influenced by them in their handling of children in hospital.

The scientist forms a *hypothesis*, that is, a general statement that he believes certain events to be connected. He then tries to think what would follow:

(*a*) if his guess were right,
(*b*) if his guess were wrong.

The experiment or scientific observation is then planned to test the hypothesis. For example, you may believe that the smell of gas you detect in a room comes from a faulty gas pipe leading to the cooker. There is, in the same kitchen, also a gas water heater and a gas ring. If the hypothesis is right turning the gas off at the main will stop the smell, turning off the cooker will also do so, but turning off the other two taps will not have any effect.

In the *experiment* to test the hypothesis one operation after the other is performed, care being taken to ensure that no unknown variables occur. If, for instance, a friend turns off the main while you are testing the oven, or if someone turns the other two taps off at the wrong moment, the experiment is spoilt.

You could, of course, carry out a different experiment; you could put a match to the supposed gas leak in the oven. This would be a suitable experiment to disprove your hypothesis if you were mistaken; but, if you were right, it would cause an explosion. It would be, from the scientific point of view, a satisfactory experiment, but one which is indefensible because of its effect.

In psychological study many experiments must be ruled out because, even if they proved the hypothesis right, they would be indefensible and unethical.

It is, for example, a hypothesis of some psychologists that children deprived of mother love grow into emotionally stunted individuals, but it is clearly impossible to carry out an experiment to prove that this is so. This is why controlled observation is a method more frequently used in psychology than experiments.

Some experiments, however, have proved possible and very profitable. It was, for instance, casually observed that some people allowed a good deal of time to elapse before responding to a visual stimulus. A number of hypotheses were formulated, for instance:

1. There is always a measurable time interval between the moment when a light is shown and when a person reacts to it by pressing a button; this is called 'reaction time'.
2. People differ in their reaction time.
3. Reaction time is slower if the individual being tested is tired or under the influence of alcohol.

If these hypotheses are true they are of interest to motorists, for example, and to pilots, and to nurses, who must react quickly to patients' signals or to danger signs.

Experiments can easily be set up to test the hypothesis. Suitable apparatus can be constructed, reaction times carefully measured, volunteers found for the experiments, care being taken that only one variable is introduced into the experiment at a time, e.g. the subject must not be hungry, cold, drunk and tired simultaneously. Books on psychology describe many interesting experiments carried out on people and animals, dealing with learning, forgetting and other mental activities, the experiments being just as carefully conducted and as valid as those in other sciences.

An interesting piece of research, often referred to as the Hawthorne experiment, was carried out in a factory to find out in what circumstances production could be increased. Five girls participated. One by one factory conditions were altered. The temperature of the room was increased, then decreased; noise was reduced, then increased; rest pauses, the seating arrangement and lighting were altered, one by one. Every single alteration in environment resulted in increased output. This experiment showed that psychologists were probably mistaken in believing that only external environment affected work to any great extent. Instead, they came to the conclusion that output rose because of the interest which was being taken in the girls' progress. The fact that change is introduced conveys to the worker the interest of management.

The findings of this experiment have led industrial psychologists into an entirely different field—that of industrial 'morale'. Psychologists are now widely employed in industry to help raise the morale of the workers. Hospitals are finding some of the industrial research very relevant.

Controlled observation is, however, the most widely used psychological method. Instead of setting up experiments designed to bring about a particular result in people, those already showing the characteristic are observed. If, for example, juvenile delinquency were to be studied no attempt would be made to create delinquents, but those who already were delinquent would be studied.

In a school every child who had been before a juvenile court might be matched with a child having no record of delinquency, efforts being made to ensure so far as possible that the two groups were alike in age, sex, intelligence, social and economic standing. Having found a suitable control group with which to compare the experimental group enquiries about the family of each child would be instituted and it might be discovered that significantly more of the delinquent group came from broken homes. This would provide one possible clue to the causation of delinquency, but the relationship would not in every case be true. There may be some delinquent children whose parents are happily married and some normally adjusted children in very unhappy homes. But, if the percentage of broken homes in the delinquent group were found to be so much greater than in the control group that it could not possibly be due to chance, the discovery would be sufficiently important to be taken into account.

A great deal of psychological knowledge has been gained by the method of comparing groups of people. There is a very high probability that children who do well in intelligence tests will do well at a grammar school; that nurses who have been selected because of their high score in a particular selection test will do well in the State Examination. There is evidence that patients suffering from gastric ulcer more often have personal difficulties than patients suffering from, say, appendicitis.

Because psychological findings apply to groups and are stated in rather cautious terms people applying psychological knowledge must be careful in the use they make of it. It is a statement of fact that many mentally disturbed people have had an extremely strict upbringing. It would be wrong to interpret this statement by saying either that all mental illness is caused by strict upbringing, or that in every case strict upbringing causes mental illness. This latter interpretation was at one time accepted and licence was advocated as the correct method of bringing up children, not by psychologists, but by those teachers or parents who had failed to understand psychological findings.

Psychologists can not be held responsible for any particular course of action taken by the public or by a professional body or individual. They might be able, for example, to show in terms of probability that flogging is likely to arouse resentment and increase, rather than decrease, violent activities. Whether or not we abolish flogging in the home and in schools as an official form of punishment must be decided by individual fathers, by teachers as a professional group and by the nation as a whole. Again, psychologists might be able to show, in terms of probability, the relationship between visiting children in hospital and the incidence of various forms of maladjustment after the child goes home. Whether or not hospitals allow or encourage visiting, and whether mothers take advantage of the facilities, must be decided by the people concerned, taking psychological findings into account.

Psychology is the Science of BEHAVIOUR and EXPERIENCE

When small infants are studied it is only possible to observe *behaviour*. We can describe the infant's crying, how long he cries, how loudly he cries, his movements, which part of the body he moves, how vigorously he moves. We can also attempt to discover which stimuli in the environment are related to the infant's response. If, for example, we put a finger in the infant's palm he closes his hand; if we put a finger into his mouth he sucks; if we stick a safety pin into his skin he cries.

We are describing a system of stimuli and responses. With care and training, and with suitable apparatus to measure muscle tension, salivation and skin resistance to electricity, we could describe stimuli and responses in considerable detail. All this is termed behaviour. Some psychologists believe that behaviour is in fact the only thing which they should study. The American psychologist, Watson, has put forward this proposition most strongly and has founded the school of 'behaviourist psychology'. Behaviourists study not only infants but also all varieties of animals, particularly rats, and have contributed a large amount of knowledge. Nurses frequently have to confine their observations to behaviour. When a patient is unconscious, or too ill to speak, his behaviour is the only thing nurses can observe and this leads the nurse to discover the stimulus which is troubling him.

On the whole, however, as nurses we would find the study of psychology dull and unrewarding if we could not include the study of experience. *Experience*, in psychological language, refers to the mental phenomena occurring directly to the individual; in Spearman's words, 'something lived, undergone, enjoyed and the like'. Thinking, feeling, seeing, hearing, wishing, planning are all 'experiences'. Experiences cannot be observed by others, they can be reported only by the experiencer.

When we stick a pin into an infant this stimulus causes the behaviour of crying. We assume he experiences pain. We cannot really say anything about his experience, but we can hardly refrain from thinking that his experiences may be similar to our own.

It is the study of experience in addition to the study of behaviour which makes psychology interesting and relevant to nursing. We are interested in what our patients and all the other people we meet in our life feel, think, suffer or enjoy and we select from the science of psychology that which helps us to understand human beings in the particular situations in which we meet them as nurses.

The Scope of the Subject

Psychologists study many more aspects of behaviour and experience than are of immediate interest to nurses. Each individual psychologist must restrict his work to one small section of the science. Some are concerned with the study of learning; some are interested in phenomena of perception, namely, the laws which govern how stimuli arriving at the sense organs are interpreted into something meaningful, how past knowledge affects perception.

Some study the behaviour of animals; others are concerned with the study of child behaviour or development; some are concerned with investigation of the effect of early childhood experiences; and others are interested in the interaction of people with each other in small and large groups. Some psychologists are interested in social phenomena, such as racial prejudice, and they try to relate these phenomena to the personality development of the people concerned; others work in industry.

The fact that psychologists differ in their interests, that there are many different ways of approaching the subject, many methods of study and many ways of presenting the findings, has resulted in various 'schools of psychology' emerging. Behaviourism, the gestalt school and analytic schools of psychology are examples of these. Some people believe that a multiplicity of schools must mean that nothing is known about psychology and that therefore everybody's guess is as good as anyone else's. This is, of course, a totally mistaken view. Different schools of psychology represent different spheres of interest and occasionally different ways of interpreting or applying the same facts. Facts there are in plenty. It is the task of the nurse to be informed of as many as possible of the facts which relate to her work and her life, to understand how these facts were established and what predictions are possible from the knowledge of these facts.

The nurse should understand the significance of the facts and the interpretation psychologists have put upon them. In her work the nurse's own interpretation and her own ability to sift, select and criticise will help her to apply what she has learnt to the best advantage.

SUGGESTIONS FOR FURTHER READING

There are many good textbooks of psychology. They are too detailed to be read in their entirety and go more deeply into the subject than some nurses may wish to go. They should, however, be consulted for reference. Some of these contain excellent illustrations. Students should note how carefully the authors quote exact references of experimental work. Here are some suggestions:

BROADBENT, D. E. *Behaviour.* New York: Basic Books, 1961.

DEESE, J. *General Psychology.* Boston: Allyn and Bacon, 1967.

HILGARD, E. S., ATKINSON, R. L. and ATKINSON, R. C. *Introduction to Psychology*, 5th ed. New York: Harcourt Brace, 1973.

KRECH, D., CRUTCHFIELD, R. S. and BALLACHEY, E. L. *Individual in Society.* New York: McGraw-Hill, 1962.

MUNN, N. L. *Psychology*, 5th ed. London: Harrap, 1966.

THOULESS, R. H. *General and Social Psychology*, 5th ed. London: University Tutorial Press, 1967.

WOODWORTH, R. S. and MARQUIS, O. G. *Psychology, a Study of Mental Life*, 20th ed. Methuen, 1963.

The following are short, simple introductory texts:

KNIGHT, R. and M. *A Modern Introduction to Psychology*, 7th ed. London: University Tutorial Press, 1966.

McGHIE, A. *Psychology as applied to Nursing*, 6th ed. London: E. and S. Livingstone, 1973.

ZANGWILL, O. L. *An Introduction to Modern Psychology.* London: Methuen, 1950.

The following deal with historical development of the subject:

BRETT, G. S. *Brett's History of Psychology* (edited and abridged by R. S. Peters). London: Allen and Unwin, 1962.

FLUGEL, J. C. *A Hundred Years of Psychology*, 4th ed. by D J. West. London: Methuen, 1970.

THOMSON, ROBERT. *The Pelican History of Psychology.* Harmondsworth: Penguin, 1968.

WOODWORTH, R. S. *Contemporary Schools of Psychology*, 9th ed. London: Methuen, 1965.

PART I

Psychology and the Patient

1. INTRODUCTION

Nursing is a very skilled job. It requires knowledge and manual dexterity, but, most of all, an interest in people and the ability to understand and help them.

The nurse meets people every moment of her working day: patients, colleagues, patients' relatives, and members of her own community whose continued good health is in some way or other dependent on her job. Some of the people she meets are old, some young, some mature, some immature, some are people whose personalities are agreeable, others have personality characteristics which make them difficult to get on with. Some behave appropriately to their age, others appear rather childish.

The nurse must carry out her nursing duties whatever obstacles other people may put in her way. Indeed, the obstacles created by others are part of the nursing task. It is futile to say that a nursing procedure could be carried out if only the patient were more co-operative. Rather it should be said that gaining the patient's co-operation or co-operating with the patient is part of the nursing procedure.

Again, it is idle to complain that junior nurses do not carry out instructions and that the senior is left to do the job herself. It is part of every nurse's job to learn how to delegate, instruct and supervise.

The relationships with others into which a nurse enters in the course of her work make her job interesting and rewarding and success in this is partly brought about by her own personality. The right kind of person often intuitively creates confidence in the patient and understands other people's needs. The personality of the nurse directly or indirectly affects the well-being of the patient. Her manner of calming an anxious relative or dealing with a disgruntled member of the lay staff will be felt indirectly by the patient.

It is, however, not possible to recruit to nursing only people who have already acquired the necessary personality and also possess all the required skills. Those who have not yet done so can learn by studying how people behave, how they differ from each other, how they develop and how their development is influenced by social pressures and environment. The study of personality is, therefore, an essential part of the nurse's preparation for her work.

Personality is the term used to describe the complex pattern of integration and interaction of psychological and physical characteristics, which make each person a unique individual. To study any one 'personality' it is necessary to acquire a detailed record of all he does, his ambitions, his wishes and desires, his thoughts, his dreams, and a knowledge of the way in which he experiences the world around him. His feelings have to be studied and also his temperament and his attitude to people and events.

All these various aspects of mental life have to be described and if possible measured. Their consistency over a period of time must be noted. The psychologist looks back over a person's life to try to understand how he came to acquire his present personality and looks forward to see where his present personality traits are taking him.

Later on we shall take another look at the study of personality and its various components. At the moment it suffices to note how complex and varied adult personality is—how simple and almost uniform, by contrast, the behaviour of the new-born infant. How the change occurs during the process of growing up is the subject matter of the next few chapters.

2. INFANCY

The most striking experience when observing a newly born infant is one's awareness of his complete helplessness. Mothers, of course, see in their own infant all the possible virtues, all perfection, all miraculous achievements. Independent observers, however, can see that the newly born infant is capable of only a very small number of actions in response to a very small number of stimuli.

An infant moves his body and limbs in a generalised, non-purposive sort of way; he is not able to carry out any precise movements of any part of his body with the exception of a very few reflex actions.

When something, a finger for instance, is placed into the palm of the infant's hand, the hand closes in a grasping movement, which is so firm that the child's whole weight could be supported by his arm. If the cheek is touched the infant turns his head towards the stimulus, a useful reflex enabling the baby to find the nipple of the breast. When the nipple, or the teat of the bottle, or the fist arrives in his mouth the infant sucks.

It is possible to make the infant cry by making sudden loud noises or by suddenly withdrawing support. Often a baby will cry when his mother passes him on to father, possibly a reaction to sudden loss of support rather than an awareness of mother's skill or father's clumsiness. After a little while in his father's arms the baby probably settles down again just as he did with his mother.

An infant may also cry in other circumstances; namely, when a pin sticks into him, when he has not been fed for several hours, when the nappy is being changed. We are apt to say then that the baby is in pain, or perhaps hungry or cold.

These statements are, strictly speaking, unjustified. It is not really possible to know what a baby experiences. Hunger, pain, discomfort are states of conscious experience which generally we can communicate to others only in words. Babies cannot speak. Their only method of communication is crying. In everyday language it is, of course, quite acceptable to attribute to the baby experiences which we believe we would have if we were short of food, had a pin sticking into us, or were wet and cold. In psychological language, however, it is worth while to distinguish clearly between 'behaviour' which can be easily observed—in this case crying—and interpretation, about which we may easily be wrong. Nurses have to do this frequently, i.e. they must observe behaviour and make tentative guesses about the patient's experience, not only with babies but with any patient who is unable to speak; such as the unconscious patient, or the patient who has lost his speech due to cerebral haemorrhage or laryngeal damage, or the patient suffering from depression or schizophrenia who will not speak.

Just as we cannot really say what an infant is feeling when he cries neither can we say how he feels when he lies awake in his cot or snugly in his mother's arms. Yet we feel that the words 'contentment', 'satisfaction', 'pleasure', 'gratification' somehow describe what it must be like to be warm, well wrapped up, rocked, securely held, adequately fed. We feel justified in talking about 'needs' which must be satisfied if the infant is to develop normally. Most infants have all their needs satisfied because the mother's needs, which are to love, comfort, support, protect and nurse, correspond completely with the needs of her infant. In the interaction between mother and infant the two are so completely at one that for the time being it is impossible to see the child as having a separate personality at all. This unity of mother and infant, the emotional and physical bond which exists at the time of birth, appears to be necessary for the infant's development.

No infant could possibly survive if he were denied all forms of care and protection. If after birth a child is denied some of the emotional warmth, love and affection most infants receive we then speak of him as being a deprived child—deprived of love and security. A mother may not have looked forward to her baby's birth, she may have resented pregnancy, or have suffered ill health during pregnancy, or she may have grown to dislike the child's father or may perhaps not even know who the father is. If her child is deformed or ugly it may be difficult for the mother to feel wholly accepting. Some mothers suffer from physical or mental disorders following childbirth and the mother's admission to hospital may make it impossible for her to give all the emotional care to her child that she may desire. For any of these reasons a child may be 'deprived'. It is now often believed that the best thing is to provide the baby with a mother substitute. Grandmother, father, neighbour, aunt or nurse can, by devotion and continued presence, satisfy the baby's emotional needs, but social workers find it difficult to assess whether the benefit of substitute care would outweigh the advantage of continued care from the child's natural parents.

In many hospitals or nurseries every endeavour is made to allow one nurse to care for the infant, for he appears to need personal care, loving, cuddling, holding, as much as food and bodily attention. He thrives best if one person gives him the whole of herself.

There is still too little evidence to show how soon after birth the continuity of care becomes essential. Some people feel that the first few days do not matter very much and that the hospital routine just after birth does not affect the infant. Others, however, believe that the mother establishes a bond with her infant right from birth, or rather that it should never be severed by removing the infant from her. For this reason delivery at home rather than in hospital is favoured by many so that a mother with help, preferably from the father, can care for her baby from the start and so that the infant never suffers from the changes in nursing staff to which some babies born in hospital are exposed. Even in hospital it is sometimes possible to keep each infant with its mother and so help the bond between mother and child to grow and strengthen.

Breast feeding is often thought to be essential to the healthy growth of the infant. During breast feeding unity between mother and infant is greatest, satisfaction of motherhood is experienced to the fullest extent, the infant is completely relaxed and satisfied. When breast feeding is established easily it provides a uniquely satisfying experience both to mother and child. If there is difficulty, however, either because the mother finds she has not sufficient milk, or the infant does not suck well, or the mother resents the infant and his demands on her time, then breast feeding is probably harmful as tension and anxiety affect both mother and child. Bottle feeding, if the baby is well held, well supported and properly nursed before, during and after feeding and if the same person nurses the baby each time, can satisfy the infant's needs while insistence on breast feeding increases difficulties.

Nurses, whose duty it is to help and advise the expectant or the younger mother, should know how important is the mother's love and care and how satisfying it is to most women to gratify the infant's need.

Encouragement and understanding help the mother to develop a healthy attitude towards her infant if her difficulties are understood and anticipated. Many young women are afraid of motherhood; afraid they may not be equal to it, that something may go wrong, or that they have made a mistake in starting a family. Some have mistaken ideas about the physiology of pregnancy, are reluctant to give up their freedom, or resentful about men and guilty about their own behaviour.

If a woman has to deal with her emotional difficulties it is not easy for her to look forward to motherhood and to welcome her child with the serene, loving acceptance which the infant requires. It may be difficult for a mother to express in words the anxieties she feels, difficult for her to understand them and even more difficult for her to communicate them to the nurse.

Some antenatal clinics arrange educational programmes, films, discussions, lectures, which aim at allaying many of the most common anxieties without giving voice to them. Yet every mother's problems, however similar they may be to those of others, are peculiarly her own and need the special understanding of the nurse. In her anxiety to do the best for the child the nurse must guard against creating guilt feelings in those women who find the new experience of motherhood too difficult at first.

In many instances the young mother seeks the advice of the nurse about the way in which she should feed and nurse her baby. If she is doing well, is happy, confident, relaxed and if the baby is satisfied, the mother, though she is asking for advice, does not really need it. She needs the approval of the nurse, the confirmation that all is going well. When the baby does not thrive and the mother is anxious she is more clearly in need of help. But, before advising her, it is well to remember that an anxious person seeks advice from as many sources as possible and is apt to obtain conflicting counsel. Moreover, in her anxiety she may not fully understand the advice given to her and only be able to follow it partially.

There is no clear-cut advice, applicable to all cases, that psychologists can offer. For example, to the questions whether to feed the infant regularly, or whenever he appears to demand food, whether to let him cry or respond to his crying by picking him up, there is no single answer.

When mother and baby are both well and attuned to each other it appears that the baby will establish a regular pattern of waking and sleeping. The pattern may not be precisely four-hourly, nor exactly at 2, 6, and 10 o'clock, but the baby will not lack all rhythm if his mother allows *him* to establish the routine. Certainly some routine appears necessary to the infant, the most important routine of all being the regular appearance of food and of mother love; comfort and food are both part of the same experience, representing the satisfaction of needs. Infants who do not establish regular rhythms of sleeping, waking and feeding may lack the sense of security which the normal mother-child relationship gives. A mother who is too anxious or too troubled to fulfil her role adequately cannot benefit from advice. She needs help in the form of a willing listener and encouragement to develop strength and confidence in her own ability as a mother.

Discussion with a nurse, who is interested but not critical, or with other mothers who have similar problems, can help a mother to gain understanding and to modify her attitude. She may recognise, for example, that her own inability to love and be loved causes her to treat her infant as if he were inanimate and refer to him as 'it' and attend too rigidly to physical care to the exclusion of an emotional relationship. Recognising her difficulty and having her own need accepted by the nurse she may be able to let her feelings develop. Some mothers become excessively attached to the infant. At the time when the infant might be ready to develop some independence the mother may become more possessive and protective in order to satisfy her own need for affection. Discussion of her problems may help her to realise the danger to the child of excessive attachment and may help her to satisfy her own emotional needs elsewhere.

Very rapidly, during the first few months, the infant's behaviour changes. New responses appear almost daily, new knowledge is acquired and the infant develops a personality of his own and his own way of influencing others. Every new achievement is greeted with joy and admiration by the mother and father and the rapidity of learning seems little short of miraculous. Yet few parents know how their infant's development compares with that of others. They measure their child's progress against their own expectations and ambitions rather than by the standards exhibited by other children. During the first few months the child's rate of progress often exceeds expectation so that many mothers are amazed to see how far advanced their babies are. Later, parents' expectations are often unrealistically high and disappointment leads to excessive pressure on the child. It may be helpful to a mother if a nurse can tell her how her own child is progressing in comparison with others. Mothers' meetings in postnatal clinics, informal gatherings of mothers in the park, or ordinary social contact between mothers all serve for the exchange of information but frequently result in great anxiety when a mother becomes aware that her own child is less advanced than a friend's and when she feels unable to express her fears or discuss her difficulty. The nurse's knowledge of many children and her awareness of the norms of development may enable her not only to reassure the mother who worries unnecessarily, but also to draw attention to delayed development which the parents may be unwilling or unable to acknowledge.

It is only relatively recently that a systematic survey of children's behaviour at various ages has been undertaken. Muscle activity has been observed in detail and development from generalised movement of the body as a whole to the detailed movement of finger and thumb has been listed, described and photographed. Development of eye movements and of posture have all been studied. Similarly, eating habits, sleep and elimination have come under scrutiny and, at a later age, the growth of social behaviour and development of thought and language. Some of these studies were carried out by Gesell, at the Clinic of Child Development, Yale University.

Table I. NORMS FOR DEVELOPMENT

Described by Arnold Gesell

16 weeks:	Eyes focus on mother or dangling toy.
	Turns head on hearing noise.
28 weeks:	Sits alone.
	Reaches out for toy.
	Grasps with palm of hand.
	Begins to articulate sounds.
40 weeks:	Can grasp toy between fingers and thumb.
	Pulls himself up and stands holding furniture.
	Imitates syllables.
52 weeks:	Creeps about freely.
15 months:	Begins to walk.
	Speaks a few words—da, no.
18 months:	Bladder control almost established during the day.

When hundreds of babies have been observed it is possible to state at what precise age 50 per cent of the babies have mastered any particular skill. The age is then taken to be the norm for the particular activity. It is an average figure obtained by taking into account the slowest and the most rapidly developing children. No parent should worry because his child's performance is below or above the average. Variations within normal limits are great. It is only when a child differs so greatly from the norm that some help is obviously required that the nurse should draw attention to it. More frequently she may have to explain to parents that norms are merely rough guides, not absolute standards of perfection.

Parents may indicate their sense of responsibility for the child's progress by asking many questions about development. They may, for instance, wish to know how much of a child's future is determined by heredity, how much by the environment they will be able to provide. They may also wish to know how actively they should help their child to learn, how much of the child's development is simply due to maturation rather than to learning.

All these are difficult questions to answer and the nurse's greatest contribution may lie in encouraging parents to express their fears and beliefs rather than in making authoritative statements.

It appears fairly certain that some hereditary factors determine personality development. Right from infancy some children are placid, others more active. Some normal children sleep a great deal, others very little. These temperamental differences are probably innate. The infant's temperament, however, determines from the very first moment how he is handled, how people feel towards him and how he, in turn, experiences his environment. Human development is so slow, experiences between infancy and adulthood are so numerous, that it is very difficult to discover how much environment has affected the individual, and how much the individual has influenced his environment.

In animals which reach maturity rapidly, and particularly in those animals which hatch after their parents' death, such as insects, or which are deserted by their parents, such as cuckoos, it is easy to see that certain behaviour patterns are non-learnt. We call them instinctive if they are universal to the whole species and cannot possibly have been learnt. The nesting behaviour of birds, the mating rituals of certain fishes, the egg-laying behaviour of some insects are clearly instinctive. There is some doubt as to whether the instinctive behaviour is always perfect and precisely the same in every member of the species. When it is not perfect the animal may not survive, so we may not be able to see imperfect examples. Improved photographic technique has established that the nearer the animal's behaviour is to its goal the more stereotyped, i.e. the more invariable, it becomes. Although the beginnings of nest building or sexual dances may vary the finishing touches of the nest or the consummatory act of sexual behaviour is invariable. The instinctive acts are carried out as specific responses to absolutely specific stimuli. The term 'innate release mechanism' has largely replaced the term 'instinct', because the point that specific stimuli result in specific behaviour is made much clearer by the former expression. Some herring-gulls, for example, peck specifically at a red spot on the mother herring-gull's beak; a pencil with this colouring pattern could evoke the same response. Some female fishes respond to the red surface on a cardboard fish even better than to the coloured undersurface of a male fish. Some birds take flight when shown a figure that resembles a hawk in flight when moving in one direction, but they remain calm when the figure moves in the opposite direction, resembling an aeroplane. There is an innate ability in animals to notice certain stimuli and to react to them.

Most behaviour in human beings is so much modified by learning that it is hardly ever possible to discover instinctive reactions. Perhaps the nearest to this form of innate release mechanism is the infant's tendency to smile when shown a round disc with a hole in it, perhaps a figure similar to that of the mother's face when she bends over the cot and smiles. Adults, too, smile at certain patterns and Tinbergen has studied what features babies, puppies, kittens and other young things have in common which evoke smiling and protective behaviour in adults. Smiling is instinctive, not an imitation of the mother. On the whole, however, the term 'instinct' is not a useful one when describing human action.

Human beings have certain emotions and sensations in common such as fear, hunger and thirst. They learn to perceive the stimuli which evoke these emotions. But the resultant behaviour of human beings varies so much that it is not profitable to look for instinctive reactions. McDougall, who tried to classify instinctive behaviour in human beings, failed to find any consistent pattern other than the emotions experienced and the tendency to pay attention to certain kinds of stimuli. He decided to talk of 'propensities' rather than 'instincts', but some of the people who read McDougall's earlier works still insist on using the term 'instinct' for the generalised and very variable behaviour of human beings who are hungry, afraid, angry, or in a state of sexual excitement. The variations in behaviour are the result of interaction between environment and heredity, making it impossible to estimate the effects of either.

Careful observation of infants has led us to pay more attention to the process of maturation. Human beings, unlike most animals, take many years to reach adulthood. During these years the body develops and changes take place in behaviour, both these following a characteristic sequence. The rate of development is partially determined by heredity; partly, however, it is affected by the extent to which the child's needs are met at each stage of development. Maturation really means 'ripening' and, just as it is possible to speed or delay the ripening of fruit by favourable or unfavourable conditions, so it is possible for human beings to be helped or hindered in their development. It is not possible to change the course, each stage must be successfully completed before the next step forward can be taken.

At each stage of development the child is able to learn a variety of skills. His actual achievements then depend on the cultural influences which have been brought to bear on him at the appropriate stage of development. On the whole it is useless to teach any particular skill before the appropriate stage of development is reached. Recent research has shown that early stimulation and teaching can have beneficial remote effects, but premature training can be wasteful and even harmful if it results in frustration and reduced motivation to learn. The child cannot be taught to speak until he has reached the appropriate stage of maturity. When he is able to learn progress depends on the amount of interest taken by his mother, on whether she speaks much or little to him, on the effect the child produces on others when he is able to speak. The kind of language he learns is obviously related to the language he hears. Educational research has shown that fluency in the use of language and the size of the vocabulary by the time the child enters school is related to the amount of speech used by the mother long before the child himself is able to speak.

When the mother understands the stages of maturation she is helped in her approach to such important matters as toilet training, weaning and feeding habits, play and education. The mother will not make excessive demands and she will give encouragement when the child is ready to learn. The rate of maturation is so characteristic of each individual that it is possible to gain some understanding of an adult's personality by enquiring when and how the main phase changes of maturation occurred. The age at which a child raises its head, sits, stands, walks, begins to speak, the way in which weaning and habit training were accomplished are significant. The speed of maturation and the ability to learn, once the appropriate stage of maturation is reached, are, to a large extent, innate. Ability to learn is often referred to as 'intelligence'. We shall later discuss more fully what is meant by intelligence and how it can be measured.

In considering child development we must be aware of individual differences in the ability of children to learn. This affects not only the manner in which the child accepts and interprets those things that are deliberately taught, but also how much he learns incidentally and how far he understands the world around him. At a very early age only those achievements which are incidentally acquired by the child are an indication of his intelligence. Those skills which any child acquires, given the opportunity and having reached the necessary level of maturity, are those which are expected of him. At an early age it is, therefore, difficult to separate 'maturation' from intelligence. Indeed, the rate of progress of maturation is an indication of intelligence. Excessively slow development should certainly cause low intelligence to be suspected and expert advice should then be sought to establish whether a physical defect or adverse environmental influence is hindering the child's development. Children who are subnormal in intelligence may retain primitive reflexes well beyond the usual age. It is important to remember that sensory deprivation may result in delayed intellectual development. This is true whether deprivation is caused by the child's handicap, such as partial or total blindness or deafness, or by an excessively restricted environment.

The new-born infant's time is largely spent in sleep. Complete relaxation during sleep is an indication that one of the infant's needs is being met. During waking hours the infant frequently shows a restless, irritable type of behaviour which may not be specific. The infant can be comforted by being fed, rocked or cuddled. Sometimes thumb-sucking comforts him. These activities satisfy other needs of the infant. He begins to discover his environment (although we cannot know for certain what the infant knows, or which of his senses he uses to learn). Ideas and impressions of the world around him gradually develop, unknown to the adults who minister to him. Conclusions about the infant's experience can only be arrived at by inference; there is no direct way of knowing how the infant feels, what he sees or hears, nor what his needs are. Careful observation and experiment allow one to judge to which stimuli the infant is responding. In order to guess which of his needs is being satisfied one observes which situation restores the infant to a relaxed state after a period of restlessness. Observation of the infant's behaviour

shows that very soon, before he reaches the breast, his
mother's touch, her voice, her footsteps seem to satisfy him.
Very soon his eyes converge. His mother believes that he can
see because his eyes follow her, follow moving lights and can
converge and apparently focus on a toy. It has been observed
that infants smile, at about six weeks, when a face in full front
view moves up and down over the edge of the cot. A cardboard disc with two holes elicits a smiling response even more
promptly. It takes several weeks before smiling becomes a
selective response to the face of the mother. Only then can we
say that the infant knows or remembers or recognises the
mother.

Some of the infant's 'learning' may be described as 'conditioning'. This is a process first demonstrated by Pavlov
using dogs. A new stimulus becomes associated with a response previously associated with another stimulus.

Pavlov showed that a dog first salivated only when it was
given food. If a bell were persistently rung before every meal
the dog began to salivate at the sound of the bell. This only
continued, however, if—at least from time to time—food
followed the bell. When, however, the bell was rung too often
without food following salivation ceased, the dog having
become 'deconditioned'. 'Reinforcement' of the conditioned
response must take place if the acquired behaviour is to remain.

The infant soon begins to suck when he is picked up,
before he reaches the breast. He stops crying at a sound from his
mother before he is fed. These are probably conditioned
responses, the earliest forms of learning. Obviously, the mother
must continue consistently to feed the baby if deconditioning
is to be avoided. The infant begins to be able to anticipate
what his mother will do. Her consistent response, her repeated appearance, her invariable ability to satisfy his needs
is what promotes 'security'.

Security is the ability to predict what will happen in the future. 'Secure employment' means that the worker can predict that he will not be sacked at a moment's notice and that he will not be long without work. He feels secure in his work when he has grasped the routine and can predict what will be expected of him. On the first day in a new job the novice feels insecure because he does not yet understand the environment in which he moves. Newly admitted patients are insecure because they do not yet know the way of life in a hospital ward. The infant is unable to understand anything about his environment. He is at first completely passive, all kinds of incomprehensible happenings go on around him. His security lies in the fact that at least one thing can be understood and relied on—his mother's love and her ability to satisfy his needs.

A child needs security throughout his development. At all stages the chief factor in feeling secure consists in being able to rely on love, affection and approval. If these remain constant the child can enjoy variable and unpredictable adventures in an unknown world.

Experiments have shown that perception by sight is very complex and difficult; and that size, distance and shapes can be meaningful only when their relationship to each other has been learnt and when other senses have been used in combination with sight. People whose sight is restored late in life have to learn to see shapes. It is unlikely that the young infant can use sight as a means of knowing about his environment though eye movements in response to light stimuli occur early.

Sight and hearing tell us about distant things whereas touch is the most immediate source of knowledge. It occurs within our own body although language tends to confuse the source of the stimulus with the awareness of it. We say that the fire is warm, but when we get too near heat and pain are manifestly felt in the skin. Knives are sharp, it is said, but in fact it has been learnt that pain is suffered in the finger when it is cut. The infant's earliest knowledge of his surroundings certainly occurs from his sense of touch, particularly in his mouth. The mouth, lips and tongue are, throughout life, very sensitive organs of touch. A slight roughness of the fingernails, for example, can be easily detected with the tongue. Very small holes in a tooth, very small ulcers in the mouth, feel quite large when explored with the tongue. Very small lumps or foreign bodies in food are easily detected. The texture rather than the taste of food often determines whether a child accepts a new food or not.

The infant's increased knowledge of his surroundings is accompanied by an awareness of his own separate identity. When he sucks the breast or bottle his sensations are in his mouth. When he sucks his own fist he has twofold sensations —in his mouth and his fist. As he begins to move about his cot, knocks his body against the sides, plays with his own limbs, puts his toes and fists into his mouth, he is learning about his own boundaries, becoming aware of his own 'body image'. For a long time to come he will develop his body image through play so that, although his size and shape are constantly changing, he is constantly aware of himself. He can use his body—any part of his body later on—and he will become aware of the continuity of his 'self' in spite of the constantly changing circumstances.

To have an accurate body image activity of the body in relation to the environment is essential. Skill in games and grace of movement are the result of accurate body image. Some children, whose movements are restricted, whose opportunity for play is curtailed, or who suffer from disorder of the nervous system have difficulty in acquiring an accurate body image. Some idea of the magnitude of the infant's task can be gained when we realise how difficult it is for adults to change their body image. A deformity or disfigurement, for example, is very difficult to accept. Patients who lose a limb or whose limb is in plaster often find it difficult to change their body image.

The infant's body is constantly changing in size, weight and ability to move, so that the growing awareness of 'self' is a slow and complicated process. He has to learn not only the physical boundaries but also how far the body image extends. It is difficult, for example, to decide when the food that has been eaten becomes part of the consumer. While in the mouth it is still separate. Does it become part of the body when it is swallowed or only when it is in the stomach or not until it is absorbed? Are faeces part of the human being?

Some psychologists believe that the process of learning to distinguish the 'self' from the 'not self' is very important in development. A very young infant cannot distinguish clearly between himself, his mother and the food she provides. It is as if the infant were taking the mother into his own body image. As he grows he perceives his own identity and separates it from his mother. Knowledge of growth and development as described in this and subsequent chapters may be helpful to nurses who have any dealings with children or with young parents. Another reason for learning about development is the belief of many psychologists that early childhood events partially determine what kind of adult personality will finally emerge. It is interesting to find out how much people remember of their early experiences. Some psychologists claim that special techniques of psychoanalysis enable people to recall events from the earliest months of life. Because the infant has no speech, no thought in terms of adult concepts, it must be assumed that his early experiences are recalled in the realm of feeling.

3. EARLY CHILDHOOD

During the first year the infant's progress is more rapid than at any other time. Careful observation of photographs and films taken at regular intervals and detailed records of behaviour are now available, showing how muscle control progresses, in what order the infant learns new movements and when co-ordination takes place between eyes, grasping movements and movements of hands towards the mouth. When this stage is reached the infant is ready to explore his environment in play.

Learning to Perceive

One of his most important achievements is his ability to oppose the thumb to the other fingers. The use of tools and fine work would be impossible without this. It has been suggested that in this ability lies the most far reaching difference between man and animals. Even in the first months after birth, the infant follows an object with its gaze and, some time before it is able to grasp the object, it reaches out and is able to turn the head to follow the object when it has gone out of its field of vision.

At about 6 months the infant is able to pick up bricks, beads, spoons or any other object within his reach and very soon he learns more about their size and texture by putting them into his mouth and by banging them to discover what noises can be made. He puts small objects into boxes, moves them about, fits them together and generally becomes familiar with the characteristics of the material world around him.

It is necessary for his development that he should be allowed to explore, not only with his eyes but by finding out what he can reach, how much effort is required and all the possible uses to which things can be put. Even the adult really knows about objects only when he has used them in various ways.

When he sees exhibits in a museum he often feels tempted to pick them up and handle them. If this is not allowed he may feel that his appreciation of the exhibit is incomplete. Men take their cars apart, boys get as much joy from assembling or dismantling toys as from playing with them. The need to find out how things can be used is ever present. The young infant's need to handle everything he sees, to bang and throw, to suck and bite must be satisfied if he is to learn and to become a lively, inquisitive child.

Learning to Conform

His curiosity is not confined, however, to harmless actions. He tries to suck things which are dirty, he throws things which are breakable, attempts to touch a fire or pull the tail of a cat. Some of his activities could be dangerous, others cannot be allowed because the objects he uses might be damaged. It becomes necessary at times to restrict the infant. The mother does this either by physically removing the object or the infant or by showing her disapproval. To avoid trouble by keeping dangerous objects such as pills, matches or pins out of the child's reach is an obvious act of child care but it is often sadly neglected.

A great deal of success in upbringing depends on the mother's skill in conveying disapproval without making the child feel that he is losing her love. The infant is learning to give up the gratification of some of his wishes in order to avoid losing his mother's approval.

Obedience to the mother's prohibitions is essential to protect the infant from dangers and the mother must give commands absolutely clearly, indicating that she means to be obeyed. Commands and firm prohibition should be given on the rare occasions when obedience can be enforced. If prohibitions occur too often, and when urgency is less compelling, it is easy to become inconsistent. Often it is easier and wiser to divert the infant's attention and bring up a new interest rather than forbid the undesirable activity. Awareness of his mother's disapproval is the infant's first step towards an appreciation of right and wrong. It can only happen if the infant is secure in his mother's love and if his compliance with her prohibitions reinforces his feeling of being loved.

Children feel very insecure if mother threatens to go away, to abandon the child in the street or to send him away if he is naughty. Such threats often fail to produce the desired effect. Instead of learning to behave more in accordance with the mother's wishes the child may learn to distrust her, or may cling excessively to her for fear of losing her. Feeding problems have been found to be associated with anxiety about the mother's withdrawal of warmth and love.

Speech

Throughout his first year of life the infant experiments with sound. The bubbling noises which delight every mother become repetitive and suddenly begin to sound like da-da or ma-ma. These sounds, of course, are instantly repeated by the father or mother who believe that the infant has uttered his first word. Parents show great delight in the child's first utterances. Their reaction to sounds which vaguely resemble words is different from their reaction to other noises. They often repeat the word after the infant who, in turn, gradually acquires the skill of repeating articulated words after the adult.

Repetition of sounds for their own sake, or in order to please the mother, is the beginning of language. Meaningful sounds develop rather slowly and there is still much research to be done to discover how children acquire the ideas which we associate with language.

In adulthood language is the main tool of communication. Often it is inadequate to convey precisely the thoughts which have been formed. Thoughts develop as they are put into words. It has been suggested that thought without language is impossible. Indeed, complex thought processes result in modification of language; acquisition of new words leads to clearer thought.

The infant's first form of communication occurs not through language but through action. Crying, gestures, expressive movement are his way of indicating his feelings. The mother communicates her feelings by caressing, cuddling, rocking, humming, singing, cooing and making general approving noises. By the time the infant has begun to articulate definite sounds (between 18 months and 2 years), his world of ideas includes his mother, knowing how to get her when he wants her, being fed, carried, rocked when he indicates his need. His first association between language and ideas concerns his own activities and his mother's reactions to his demands. He may, for instance, learn to say 'more' or 'up', or use a variety of sounds recognised by his mother only, usually expressing something he wants to do or needs from her. His first words are very often nonsense words.

Mothers often point out an object and begin to tell the child what it is. There is no evidence, however, that the child means the same object or any object at all when he uses the word. 'Spoon', for example, may stand for eating; 'bed', for going to bed; 'pussy', for 'I want to catch this', or 'I am afraid of this'. When pictures are given titles the child may mean to say he wants to sit on his mother's lap looking at a picture. Objects are very difficult to name because the same object is rarely presented in the same way. The visual impression of any object differs according to distance or the angle at which it is perceived. Its texture is different when dry or wet, it may feel warm or cold to touch, part of it may be rough, part smooth. It may take a very long time before any particular object assumes an identity and much longer before a word can be attached to it.

Even when the child has acquired considerable fluency in the use of language words are not necessarily used to communicate. They may constitute an accompaniment, in sound, to the child's actions or perceptions. Piaget calls this use of language 'egocentric'.

Some words express concepts which are so difficult that it is miraculous that the child ever understands. How, for instance, can he understand the word 'dog'? It may be anything that runs, or barks or growls, or has a tail to pull, or anything that has four legs. How can a child understand that alsatians and spaniels are both dogs? There is hardly any similarity between the two. Other mammals may look much more like dogs, yet have different names. How can the picture of a dog possibly be connected with the real animal in the infant's own home? Names are often given generalised meanings; for example, 'bus' may be anything that moves. The process of discovering when a certain word is used by others is essential to learning language. This is still done when the new languages of medicine or the more specialised concepts of particular sciences are learnt in adult life. The child makes many mistakes when he starts using words, but only by practising words can he make them his own and use them in communication.

Those who are speaking to young infants may use single words, but very soon adults begin to talk to children in complete sentences and they then pick up whole phrases. The child imitates and understands intonation but he is often totally unaware of the individual words involved in any particular phrase. His misunderstandings and mispronunciations are often very amusing. Sometimes they do not become obvious until the child learns to write or read.

When the child has learnt to pronounce words he begins to enjoy using language. He repeats all he hears, talks to himself or any audience he can find and begins to widen his vocabulary by asking questions. He appears to be very inquisitive at this time, but a little observation shows that the questions may not be as searching as they appear to be at first. He rarely listens to the answer and no answer really satisfies because the question is not meant to be interpreted too literally. He may, for instance, ask for names. This is partly a way of keeping the adult's attention, partly it is an experiment with sound. New words are joyfully accepted. Partly this represents an attempt to find out how many things have the same name, or what the word stands for.

When the question 'why' begins the child is rarely able to understand the relationships of cause and effect. He is not really asking for a cause—he is trying to express his surprise at observing something new and unexpected. The more involved the explanation by the parent the more the child repeats the question 'why'. It would be more satisfactory to ignore the grammatical form in which the question is asked and instead of answering 'because' simply discuss or give a commentary on the fact raised by the child. For a very long time the child has difficulty in understanding words which express relationships in time and place, or in cause and effect. Words like 'tomorrow', 'yesterday', 'inside', 'outside', 'I' and 'you' are confusing because they keep changing their meaning.

One little boy, for example, who was told, 'Tomorrow we go to see granny' asked: 'Is today tomorrow?' Children refer to themselves by their own name, which they often hear, rather than use the word 'I'. 'Johnnie wants a sweet', for example. The answer to 'Do you want an apple?', for example, may well be 'You want an apple' instead of 'I want an apple.' It is also very difficult for him to understand what happens to things when he cannot see them. Children often cover their eyes and think that nobody can see them. The child's difficulty in understanding the meaning of time and his inability to realise the continued existence of things which are not in sight must be remembered when the effects of separation from the mother are considered. Toddlers need their mother's presence all the time. During play they periodically return to her, or they cry to bring her back when she is out of the room.

When the mother goes away to have another baby, for example, or into hospital, or when the child has to be admitted to hospital, the one secure factor in the child's life—his mother's presence—is suddenly removed. He cannot understand the future. Assurances about tomorrow, or soon, are useless. He cannot believe in his mother's existence when she is not there and he believes himself to be lost. He feels that his mother has lost or abandoned him. Separation of the small child from the mother should be avoided whenever possible. It may not always be possible, but we shall later discuss whether it may not be sometimes advisable to keep a sick child at home rather than admit him to hospital and whether home confinements rather than hospital confinements may not be preferable from the point of view of the older child.

Some children begin to speak rather later than others. This may not have any serious significance if the child appears to develop normally in other ways and is not unhappy. Some children omit altogether the period of babbling meaningless sounds, of baby talk or repetition of single words. When they begin to talk they surprise everybody with their clear articulation, large vocabulary and accurate grammar. It may be that they practise silently or when they are unobserved. There are, however, many reasons for delay in speaking which should be investigated.

Some children manage to communicate without speech so well that they do not find it necessary to use it. Position in the family can affect speech development in a variety of ways. Older children may learn to speak early because the mother has plenty of time to speak to them. Younger children may learn more slowly, often because their mother is busy and has less opportunity to speak to them. On the other hand the reverse may happen, older children may find they can prolong babyhood and retain their mother's attention by not speaking; younger children may learn more rapidly if the older children help to teach. The words used in communication constitute only one part of the total message which passes between people. Tone of voice, gestures, intonation provide the rest. Occasionally the words convey a different meaning from the tone of voice. Mother, for example, may call the child 'darling' yet indicate by her intonation that the child is not very dear to her at that moment. Children may sometimes have difficulty in learning to speak because of the conflicting messages they receive, or they may learn to respond to tone of voice rather than to the words, for example, if the child fails to comply with instructions until the mother shouts.

Children whose general development is slow and whose intelligence is below normal begin to speak rather late. If the child makes no attempt to repeat words or play with sounds by the time he is 2 or 3 years old his intelligence should certainly be investigated. Some children are slow to learn to speak simply because no one takes the trouble to speak to them. The mother may be too preoccupied with the physical care she gives the child to think about speaking to him. If she does not love him or is afraid to show any affection she may treat the infant as if he were a doll without realising how necessary her speech is to him.

Children learn to speak sooner if they have an opportunity of hearing speech at face level. The child, who is held on mother's arm while being spoken to, or while mother sings songs or nursery rhymes, associates speech with all the other pleasant experiences of being loved and nursed. Speech from a distance does not seem to become significant to the child.

Children who grow up in institutions are in much greater danger of not learning to speak at the proper time. At home a child hears the same sounds made repeatedly by the same person. There is consistency in tone of voice, in vocabulary and in the occasions when certain words are used. In hospitals or children's homes a great number of nurses may be attending to the child, all of them too busy to speak, or, if they do speak, unable to provide the necessary repetition.

Nurses who care for small children, or who help mothers with their difficulties, need to know the importance of speaking often to these children making sure that the child learns to associate words with all his activities. When the child begins to speak he should be encouraged by being given a quicker and more accurate response to his needs than if he has to try to make them known without speech. Children love to play with adults who sing nursery rhymes to them, help them to repeat verses, and tell stories which have striking repetitions of words. They insist that precisely the same words be used on every occasion and gradually begin to join in at appropriate points. Mothers who read to their children, tell them stories and sing songs to them, teach them rhymes and give them books to play with, help their children to acquire, even early in life, a vocabulary which enables them to learn faster and make greater progress later on at school. It has been shown that children who are deprived of this opportunity early in life have a relatively small vocabulary during school years.

Among the children who do not learn to speak are, unfortunately, some who are deaf or partially deaf. Deafness is extraordinarily difficult to detect during the first two years of life. Often failure to articulate is the first indication that all is not well. Deafness is a great handicap to development. Some children have been thought to be defective and were later discovered to be deaf. Hearing aids, where possible, and special help from speech therapists and special schools are necessary to help the child to develop with a minimum amount of difficulty.

Toilet Training

During the first year of life elimination occurs automatically. Bowel action depends on the food the child is taking and on his general health. Sometimes, while the infant has chiefly milk, bowel action is so regular that observant mothers manage to prevent nappies being soiled, but as soon as mixed feeding begins, or whenever the infant is slightly unwell, bowel action becomes irregular. Toilet training is not possible until sphincter control is established and until the child is able at least to understand if not use language.

The bladder empties by reflex action whenever it is full and learning can only begin when the child can learn to recognise fullness of the bladder and communicate to someone his need for help before reflex emptying occurs.

Most people learn to control bowel and bladder at some time during childhood. The anxiety so many parents experience in their attempt to speed up control is quite irrational. Because parents believe that they should train their children in toilet habits as soon as possible they show strong emotional reaction to the child's elimination. When the child is constipated his mother becomes worried. She is pleased when the bowels function properly yet upset when the child makes a mess or plays with faeces. These emotional reactions are difficult for the young child to interpret.

Very soon the infant realises that it is in his power to influence his mother's reaction by his elimination. It is believed by some psychologists that the infant comes to regard his faeces as a product of his own which is his to give or retain as he pleases. However hard his mother may try to influence the child's natural functions he cannot be forced to give up faeces or to conform to rules and he may experience his first victory, his first awareness of independence, in relation to elimination.

Some mothers show disgust at the sight or smell of faeces and cause the child to have a feeling of guilt associated with bowel action. When toilet training begins the infant may fail to understand the mother's intentions. Sitting on a pot for long periods may be fun or may be a most unpleasant experience, but may remain totally unconnected with micturition or with defaecation.

The child may not understand why his mother is sometimes pleased when he passes urine and at other times the reverse. The association between place and action of elimination can only be formed if it is possible to make the two events coincide. Generally it has been found that children are clean soon after nappies are left off, because at that moment it becomes possible to catch the child in the act of elimination and to sit him on the pot at once. It is easier to train a child in the summer months and much easier when he is able to talk.

Bedwetting often occurs for some time after training has been established in the daytime. This is partly due to the very long night and it may help to pot the child late in the evening. Usually the child wets at the moment of waking. When he moves from cot to bed and is old enough to get out and reach the pot by himself he usually begins to have a dry bed and is proud of it.

There is no need to worry if a child is later than is usual in establishing toilet training. Psychologists believe too rigid toilet training to be positively harmful. Frequently the child reverts to enuresis later in childhood. It is also very possible that personality characteristics such as stubbornness, meanness, rigidity in outlook may be derived from the attitudes acquired in relation to elimination.

Enuresis or encopresis may have organic causes, in which case a doctor should be consulted. Excessively deep sleep may prevent waking when the bladder is full. This may occur even in adults. Drugs to reduce depth of sleep are sometimes prescribed or other methods may be used to assist waking.

The Family

Close relationship between mother and infant is so important that we have mentioned the need of it in every chapter; later capacity to love, to experience deep and warm emotion depends on it. Only in the security of love is it possible to explore the environment and learn about the complexities of life. The mother's love and approval make it possible for the child to give up gratification of some wishes and to learn to adapt his behaviour to the demands made by society.

The father enters the child's world in at least two different ways. The first experience may be of the father as a person who takes the mother away. The infant may feel jealous of the attention his mother pays to his father and may resent his presence. Awareness of the existence of a group of three people may in later life affect the attitude adopted to other triangular situations. The way in which the child copes with his feelings of resentment and jealousy of his father may be very important in his sexual development. We shall discuss this more fully in a later chapter.

The father very soon becomes an important person in his own right. He may establish a rhythm for the child's day; bedtime, meals, play, story telling, outings may all be associated with the father's presence. The regularity of events with which he is associated may become a factor in providing security. The mother may feel that the father sees the child only in favourable circumstances. He is spared participation in the many frustrating conditions which make up the mother's day. She may feel that it is unfair that the child should feel only love and admiration for his father, while inevitably feelings of hate are frequently aroused towards her because she is responsible for maintaining order and establishing discipline.

Sometimes the mother may be tempted to lay the restrictions she places on the child at the father's door: 'Wait until your father comes home', or 'Don't make a noise; father is tired', may be her way of associating the father with the idea of authority and of retaining the child's love.

Love and Hate

Many mothers find it difficult to understand how strong a child's emotions can be and how vigorously and promptly these emotions are expressed. A feeling of anger, resentment or hate is quite natural when the child is thwarted and the stronger his love for his mother the deeper the feeling of anger against her when frustration occurs. Feelings of hatred and anger are very frightening, but the child can be helped to learn to manage his emotions by his mother's understanding and acceptance. When he is aware that his mother still loves him and is still in command of the situation this helps him to gain self-control and to lose the terror of his own temper. If the child is made to feel guilty, wicked and unloved he cannot learn to control his feelings; instead he learns to hide them. He may become docile and polite, but full emotional development may later become more difficult.

The father's frequent appearance, regular play, friendly interest help the child to tolerate periods of separation from his mother. It has often been noticed that the child is angry with his mother, but not with his father, after an enforced removal from home.

Younger brothers or sisters may sometimes be the next people to enter the child's world. If the infant is less than 18 months old it is extremely difficult to prepare him for the event. Before the age of 3 years the appearance of a new infant simply means separation from the mother and a feeling of being neglected and unloved because she devotes time to the little brother or sister. However clearly the mother may know that love is infinite and indivisible the child believes that there must be less love to spare for himself if the new baby receives some of his mother's love. The child's resentment is shown in his behaviour both to his mother and to the new-born baby. At times hostility to the newborn can entail physical danger and the mother's protective attitude increases the infant's resentment against her. In order to regain her attention the older child may become more babyish in his behaviour. He may again wet and soil his pants or bed, may suck his thumb, cry or whine and generally behave like the younger child. Extra attention and care may quickly reassure him and help him to enjoy the companionship of his sibling. (This word is used to denote a brother or a sister.)

The emotional turmoil of the first few years of life finds expression in the stories which the child makes up for himself or to which he likes to listen. In his play, too, he gives vent to his feelings. The treatment meted out to a doll often gives an indication of the fate which the child would like his siblings or parents to suffer. He may solve some of his problems of family living by inventing 'dream companions' with whom he has lively discussions. He can escape from the harsh reality of his real family by creating a phantasy family of his own, which he can order about to his own liking.

Play

In an earlier chapter reference was made to the child's need to play. The infant plays with his fingers and toes, arms and legs and thus gets to know about his own body. He plays with every object he handles and learns about the material world in which he lives. As he grows older he uses most of his energy in the active exploration of his environment. He grows in strength and develops neuromuscular co-ordination in the process of playing, climbing, jumping, gymnastics of all kinds and all this is essential to his physical development and thoroughly enjoyable to him.

As he plays he meets many new and strange situations. Whenever he feels unsafe or startled he rushes back to his mother whose love and support provide the security he needs for his explorations. Children who lack love and security play much less vigorously and with less inventiveness and variety. The psychologist Harlowe has shown that the same holds true of monkeys. Only those monkeys who at least had a substitute mother in the form of Turkish towelling played freely. They rushed to the towel-mother and vigorously rubbed against it whenever they were startled by unexpected noises or movements. Monkeys reared without any substitute for their mothers remained apathetic and inactive although surrounded by play material. It is clear that the basic needs are closely related to each other. The need to play, to be active and to satisfy curiosity depends on fulfilment of the need to be secure.

During play the child begins to discover not only the physical characteristics of his environment but also the feelings of the important people in his life. In his play and in his demand for stories he tries to come to grips with emotional difficulties. The stories which he enjoys most at an early age are tales of good and bad characters, fairies and witches, bad people and good children, stories in which his growing ideas of moral values are clearly thought out and good always triumphs. The sameness of the stories, the rituals, the repetitive intonations all contribute to the child's security.

Ritual plays an important part in the child's life. There are fixed rules for almost every activity. Bath, meals, bedtime stories, dressing and undressing, tucking in and good-night kisses must all conform to the daily pattern. The child is learning the rules of life and needs a rigid framework within which to move.

At the same time there is little difference between phantasy and reality. The child's play consists in animating the environment, surrounding himself with imaginary playmates with whom conversation is sustained. The adult world of material objects is still unknown. So when he calls an upturned chair a car or a boat he is not pretending—this, to him, is absolutely real. Adult models of cars or boats may not even be recognised as such. As the child plays ordinary objects which surround him, for instance boxes, cups, saucepans, garden tools and tins, provide him with endless material for amusement and learning. Water, sand, plasticine and later paint and clay are essential play materials which permit expression of feeling, creative activity and satisfying sensations.

Not until the end of the third year is companionship with other children needed or appreciated. Before that the toddler plays alone or alongside others, but there is no co-operative effort. During the fourth year of life children begin to take notice of each other, respond to each other's needs, communicate with each other and begin to enjoy social intercourse.

Although the child's play is still very egocentric mutual help is often given. Bigger projects can now be undertaken. Large objects can be moved or lifted by joint action, group activities, such as organised party-games, sing-songs and tug-of-war, are now enjoyed. The child is beginning to learn that it is necessary at times to give way to others. When there are several children in the family early social experiences are provided at home. If there is no opportunity to play with other children at home, as in the case of an only child, and when no suitable playmates can be found in the neighbourhood, much benefit can be obtained from attendance at a nursery school.

Day nurseries and nursery schools have come under severe

criticism because it was felt that young children needed their mother's continuous presence and should not be separated from her for long periods of the day. By the age of 3 or 4 years, however, the intelligent, active child needs the companionship of other children and thus to be provided with more outlet for his energies than he can be allowed in his home. In recent years the importance of providing nursery schools has been rediscovered, particularly for those children who lack companionship in the home, who, because of housing difficulties, are deprived of adequate space for exploratory play, and for those whose parents are unable to provide the necessary stimulation for constructive play. By attending a nursery school for a few hours a day the child becomes used to being away from his mother for short periods and has the opportunity of using suitable play material which cannot always be provided in the house. He stays at the nursery school for much shorter hours than is necessary when real school starts and he learns social adaptation before the more serious change to school life begins. Teachers in nursery schools function to some extent as mother substitutes. The child's attitude to his nursery school teacher provides a gradual transition to the later approach to school teachers.

Role-playing games become important. Children take it in turns to play the part of mother, father, baby, doctor, nurse and patient, or, later on, teacher and child. Not only do they learn in this way to co-operate, to understand each other's point of view, to settle quarrels and differences of opinion, to fight and make peace and generally live with each other, but they also begin to appreciate the feelings and experiences of adults. The child's desire for power finds an acceptable outlet; reversal of roles gives practice in learning to accept power in others.

Throughout life we ascribe to people certain roles we wish them to play in life and we have fairly well-defined ideas of the kind of behaviour befitting each role. We think of police-men as powerful, just, incorruptible; of professors as brilliant, benevolent, absent-minded. Certain characteristics appear to be essential to each role, some are permissible but not essential, others are incompatible with it. Motherhood, for example, entails loving kindness and consideration towards children as an essential part of the role. Neglect, cruelty, disinterest, prolonged absence are incompatible with the role of a mother. In role-playing games children interpret and learn what is expected of a mother and other grown-up people. When they become the mother in the game they behave towards the children in the way in which they think the mother should behave. The children, in the game, are bathed, fed, taken for walks, put to bed. They are also scolded and punished, often very severely. This is not an imitation of mother's behaviour towards them, but an attempt to understand the mother's anger and the punishment she gives. It is at the same time a way of accepting the mother's standards and making them their own, and a method by which the child learns to cope with feelings, to express his own fears and anxieties and to be-come sensitive to other people's feelings. In the game children are much more exacting, much stricter and more punitive than their parents ever are. The standards they set for each other are infinitely higher than their parents' standards and their wrath much more uncontrolled. In reversing roles they learn how it feels to do things which usually are done to them-selves and they change the actions in the game to make re-sponses more and more realistic.

Mother and child games may become very detailed and complicated as the child becomes more and more familiar with the mother's real life: cooking, shopping, housework, concern for the father and for other children, the need for order and cleanliness, preparations for visiting—all these become part of the child's reality and are associated with the mother role. The fascination of dressing up is an important aspect of role-playing games. When the child wears different clothes he feels that he is a different person.

Other people who enter into role-playing games are never as well known as mother and children. Acquaintance with them is restricted to a particular situation; shopkeepers are only known to sell goods. What they do with the rest of their time never becomes known to the child. In much the same way fathers may only have the function of going out and coming back. What they do at work remains a mystery. They may be entitled to special privileges because they work, but their duties and responsibilities cannot be rehearsed in play.

If role-playing games are thought of as a preparation for life it is easy to see that children's preparation for life may remain inadequate. Adulthood in games consists largely of the right to tell other people what to do and not oneself having to obey. Work consists of going out and coming back; parenthood largely of privileges and only to a small extent of duties. Adults who enter into role-playing games can help considerably in preparing the child for the role he will be expected to play. By adding detail and realism to the part played by the adults one can help to prepare the child for the fact that growing up brings with it increased duties as well as increased scope. Role-playing games continue until well into school age. The parts played by each child become more complex and often more carefully scripted and rehearsed. They continue to take the child a little way ahead and thus prepare him for the next phase.

Before the child goes to school it is advisable to initiate 'school games'. Before admission to hospital each aspect of hospital life could be played out so that the child enters a familiar routine and understands the part each person in hospital has to play. The hospital game may have to be played many times, in different ways, with the child acting patient, doctor, nurse, matron, visitor. Many likely events and attitudes are thoroughly understood and anticipated and the child's fear and anxiety are recognised and conquered. Hospital games may continue for some time after the child's discharge from hospital. He may try, in the game, to convey to his mother his emotional turmoil while ill. He may relive the anxieties he experienced about all the frightening events and the fears he endured of being forgotten by his parents.

At school role-playing games are used as a means of much factual learning. Games of shopping may involve valuable arithmetic lessons, for example. Knowledge gained in this way about people continues to make acting valuable, whatever other information may be involved. Even as adults, role-playing may be a useful device for preparing for forthcoming ordeals. Examinations become less terrifying as experience in taking them is gained and may well lose much of their terror when the candidate has acted as examiner to others. This is an activity which student nurses would be well advised to carry out. Acting the patient, during practical nursing procedures, is invaluable in learning to anticipate the patients' reactions to the real thing. Playing at applying for jobs, being interviewed, interviewing and selecting others is generally a practised technique in the preparation for administration.

As the child grows older the characteristics of play change. Before the child goes to school it does not distinguish between work and play. The small girl who dresses her doll, washes dolls' clothes, or helps her mother to bake a cake, puts intense effort and concentration into what is play at the time but will soon become work. The child's absorption in a construction game, or in painting or woodwork is indistinguishable from later attitudes to work. Many lifelong interests have their origin in the enjoyable experiences of childhood play. When the child goes to school play becomes a relaxation from work associated with the more serious aspects of life, purposive yet subject to fewer external rules and restrictions than work.

Real group games now become important. At first they are usually games like 'cops and robbers'; a few years later these are replaced by organised games such as football, cricket, hockey. In these games the child learns the rudiments of the rules and standards of the adult world. Piaget has shown that children have some difficulty at first in distinguishing between different types of rules. If they are shown how to play a game (in Piaget's example, a game of marbles) they accept the rules as absolute and become indignant at the suggestion that rules can be changed. Later when they play team-games at school they can understand that the rules of the game are simply social agreements, convenient ways of arriving at co-operative effort and subject to change when all players agree. They understand the difference between 'social rules' and 'moral rules' which cannot be changed. Group games are thought to be valuable in providing an opportunity for learning moral rules. Cheating at games, for example, is not allowed; 'playing the game' means competing in a friendly way; 'it is not cricket' means it is unfair. Children learn to lose without being upset, to admire achievement in others and to submerge their own interests in the interest of the team.

When children meet difficulties in their development they often express this through play. An observant mother knows from the way her child treats her doll that she is hurt or upset. Children's moods are often reflected in their painting. Pictures tend to be all dark and grey when all is not well at home; they are brilliantly coloured and full of sunshine when the painter is happy; sometimes very red when the child is angry. The fact that play expresses so well what the child may feel while words may not easily come to him has led to play therapy as a form of treatment for severely disturbed children. Observation of a child at play with a doll's house may help one to diagnose where the problems lie; for example, in the play the baby doll may be thrown out of the window or the mother doll may have pins stuck into her. The child's comments about his painting, or even the painting itself, may help one to understand the problem. In the painting, for example, the family may be inside the house except for the child who is left outside—an indication, perhaps, of the child's loneliness and sense of exclusion from the family.

In play therapy the child is encouraged to play freely in whatever way he likes provided, of course, that he is safe. The presence of a kind, helpful, accepting adult helps the child to feel safe, and as he acts out his problems he begins to understand them. He learns to act out his emotions freely, yet safely, in the playroom. Instead of hiding his anger about his baby sister he can safely be angry in play and learn how to control his emotion in real life. In the play therapy room he is free to play with material with which he may have wished to play earlier in life but was prevented. Water, dirt, mud may not have been allowed because of his mother's excessive desire for cleanliness. In play therapy these materials are safe and permitted and however childishly he uses them he need not fear any ridicule or criticism. Finger painting provides an exciting alternative to mud or dirt. The emotional release which accompanies play and the improvement in the child after he has obtained satisfaction from play show how basic a need is involved.

Stages of Development

There are many ways of approaching the study of child development. Some observers have made specific contributions to our knowledge of physical, especially neuromuscular, development, others have paid attention to intellectual development. Some psychologists have taken a special interest in the emotional development of the child and others in the personality characteristics which are laid down in childhood. Although it is well understood that development is a continuous process psychologists tend to speak of *stages* of development and to describe the characteristics or norms of each stage. There is a considerable overlap and rarely any sudden transition.

Piaget, for example, uses the child's intellectual development as a basis for his description of stages. At first, until approximately the age of 2 years, he describes a stage of *adualism*, during which the child learns to distinguish between 'self' and 'not-self' and to build up the idea of people and objects outside himself. The next stage, from 2 to 5 years, is the stage of *animism* or *magical thinking*, in which the child's ideas about the world are unrealistic. He sees himself as the centre of the world and has no idea of the limits of his power. He enjoys making things happen, but he cannot understand the laws of cause and effect and may believe he has magical powers. Objects and people alike are seen to have feelings, wishes and desires. Everything is alive and there is no clear distinction between phantasy and reality.

Freud describes mainly stages of emotional development. In the first year the child appears to derive emotional gratification from the use of the mouth, by sucking and later by biting. Freud calls this the *oral* stage. In the second year, during the so-called *anal* stage, elimination becomes an important source of satisfaction. Then, between 2 and 5 years, Freud refers to the *genital* stage, the period when the child gains pleasure from the exploration of his body and when both boys and girls discover their sexual roles by identification with the parent of the same sex.

Erik Erikson describes the stages of development in terms of 'developmental tasks'. He points out that the child's physical, intellectual, social and emotional ability at various ages and stages determines what happens to him, what experiences he has. The way the child copes may affect the personality traits which are laid down.

In the first few months the infant is helpless. He can only wait, passively, until his needs are met. At this stage it is his task to learn to deal with 'dependency-needs'. If his needs are promptly satisfied he learns to expect that help is easily obtainable. If his needs often remain unsatisfied he may learn to develop a pessimistic outlook on life. The basic personality traits of *trust* and *mistrust* are laid down at this stage.

When the infant begins to move and to deal actively with objects and people, when he becomes aware of his identity and his ability to oppose the wishes of his mother, his task consists in developing *autonomy* and later *initiative*. Encouragement and success may help to lay down these positive personality traits. The inevitable difficulties which arise in the process of becoming autonomous may prove to be overwhelming and an attitude of *doubt* or *shame* may develop.

When the infant believes himself to be powerful he may develop a sense of *guilt* accompanying events of which he is not in fact the cause, but of which he may well imagine himself to be the cause. It may be particularly difficult for the child at this stage to be separated from his mother, because his occasional wish to be rid of her results in overwhelming guilt. In the event of the death of a parent the child may imagine that his thoughts are responsible. He may feel that he has created the marital conflicts of which he may occasionally become aware.

By about the age of 5 years a stage of development has been reached when the child has dealt with all the important tasks of infancy. Piaget describes the next stage as the stage of *realism*, while Freud talks of the *latency* stage, when feelings of emotional conflict subside. Erikson says that in the next stage the child develops basic attitudes about work, the *enjoyment of industry*, or the feeling of *inferiority* if things go wrong.

In the preceding chapter it was shown that interplay between the child and its environment is necessary for harmonious growth and development. By using its sense organs the child becomes aware of stimulation from the environment; play and exercise of all parts of the body enable it to develop dexterity. Body image and awareness of self depend on the interplay between the child and the people and objects surrounding it. A warm protective environment facilitates emotional growth; intellectual development is enhanced by a stimulating environment.

When the nurse is concerned with a handicapped child, she should remember how far-reaching the consequences of the child's disability may be, and she should do her utmost to compensate for the opportunities of which the child is deprived.

The paralysed child for example should have toys brought within reach and also be moved around to familiarise itself with different perspectives and with distance and size.

The child who cannot bring its body into contact with the surroundings needs tactile stimulation of all parts of its body.

All children need to see the world from below and above, from front and back. The child should not remain in bed or in the chair for too long, but should also lie on the floor and be lifted high up. It needs the sensation of fast movement, of turning and whirling around. No matter how slow speech development, it needs to hear the sound of words, and preferably also the sound of music, of traffic, of objects dropping to the floor, of broken glass and of clanging metal.

It is very easy to stop speaking to the child when there is

no response, but this is harmful to the child and the nurse should remember to accompany her nursing activities with the same kind of continuous chatter and commentary as that to which the normal child is exposed.

Handicapped children may pass the usual milestones late and it may seem difficult to the nurse to play with a big 5-year-old child in the manner in which she would play naturally and spontaneously with a younger child, but it has been shown that such play is necessary and that development accelerates in all areas if special attention is given to play and to speech.

4. SCHOOL

In this country the child is thought to be ready for school at about the age of 5 years. In those countries where school begins later, attendance at nursery school is much more common than it is in the United Kingdom. On starting school the child enters an entirely new phase of development.

Learning facts and skills is only a very small part of the child's new life. By far the most important aspect of school life is the social learning which it provides. For many children this may be the first time they have been obliged to submit to discipline imposed by someone other than their parents or other members of the family. Authority suddenly becomes dissociated from those the child loves most and, often for the first time, the child sees that parents are subjected to the same kind of rules as he is. Many parents still retain their fear of and respect for teachers and readily convey this fact to their children. What the teacher says suddenly becomes much more important than what the mother says. There are times when small children find their dual loyalties to teacher and parents very confusing. Small children cannot understand half measures or compromise. To the child people are either good or bad, right or wrong. It is impossible to believe that the teacher may sometimes be right, the mother at other times. As the child begins to accept the teacher's authority he may become critical, defiant and badly behaved at home.

His account of what a teacher has said is not always accurate; nevertheless, his mother may believe what he says about the teacher, may blame the school for deterioration in the child's behaviour at home and may become resentful of the school. It may be difficult to discuss fully with the teacher what the problems in the home are; parent-teacher contact may be rare and the parents' critical attitude to teachers may in turn result in the teachers' hostility towards parents. When antagonism occurs between school and home it is created by the child who exploits the situation, enjoying the fact that parents and school feel possessive about his person. Yet lack of co-operation and understanding between home and school may leave the child bewildered, unable to settle down to work and may begin an ambivalent attitude to authority which may hamper adjustment throughout life. Parent-teacher associations can help to establish co-operation between home and school if the problems are clearly understood.

Parents, friends, aunts and uncles can help the child in the difficult stage of transition by taking an interest in all that he chooses to tell them about school without prying, criticising or belittling him. Many of the child's activities at school are never discussed at home. It is important to the child to have, for the first time, a life of his own about which his mother need not know everything. Though he enjoys sharing his experiences with his mother it makes him feel big and important to be able to keep something back.

Relationships with other children at school are very different from those of the nursery years. For the first time the child's work and performance are judged on their merits and compared with those of other children. The teacher's approval is related to good work or good behaviour. At home the child is loved simply because he happens to be the child of his parents. Love is not conditional on performance, however much love and approval may be associated with conformity to rules. At home the standards set for the child are not competitive. Allowances are made for age, for feeling unwell, tired or cross. At all times the child at home is in a very special position. At school he is merely one of a large number of children treated as equals by the teacher until they prove to be otherwise. Experience of an independent figure of authority who treats all children in the same way is closely connected with appreciation of justice. Justice means that no exception is made of anyone, not even of oneself.

During the first years at school the child learns to form real friendships. Playmates before school age are rarely of the child's own choice. At school it becomes of the utmost importance to make special friends. In the characteristic way of young children a 'best friend' is found who lasts a few days and then becomes a 'worst enemy'. Friendships at this early age are completely exclusive, guarded with jealousy and bought by special favours. The criterion for the choice of a friend varies rapidly; the best behaved may be chosen one day, the naughtiest the next. Then may come the turn of the one with the nicest books or pencils, or the one who has talked about his home or his dog. Topics of conversation between friends are great secrets and the shared secret becomes the symbol of friendship.

These short-lived friendships form a valuable experience for later, more stable relationships. Because friends invite each other home, meet each other's parents, borrow each other's books or toys, the child's experience of the world expands beyond his own family circle. The other child's possessions may appear to be much more valuable and other children's parents much more exciting than the child's own. Sometimes parents reciprocate this feeling and may tend to think all other children are better behaved and much nicer than theirs. They have little idea how angelic their own offspring can be when away from home. Sometimes, of course, children who are well-behaved at home have difficulties in adjusting at school. Many people would consider it to be the main function of school to teach basic subjects; such as writing, reading and arithmetic. In fact this is only a small part of the school's purpose. Teachers would prefer not to feel that their main task was to teach these subjects, but that they were learnt incidentally. The essence of modern methods of education is that opportunity and incentive for learning are provided at all stages and that learning is an active process of the child rather than of the teacher.

The older outlook of impressing the child with the seriousness of learning led to a division in children's thoughts between work and play, between the unpleasant burden of learning and the carefree enjoyment of out-of-school activities. Modern schools maintain that learning is pleasurable and that children are more than anxious to acquire knowledge if it is presented in an interesting way at the right time. There may be practical difficulties in presenting to all children at all times interesting information of just the right sort, especially if classes are too big. If the teacher is successful, however, he may well help the child to seek knowledge and to enjoy work throughout life. Children vary in intelligence and in social maturity. Not all children are ready to learn the same things by the same method when they first enter school.

Later on it is still common practice in some schools to 'stream' classes in such a way that the children in the same form benefit from competition with each other. In the earliest years it is more common to encourage each child to work at his own rate at whatever subject interests him most. It may be more difficult for the teacher if each child in the class reads a different page in the book but it is more rewarding in the long run.

Small children cannot sit still for long and learn best if they are allowed to be generally active. Reading and writing are learnt more easily if large cards are handled, sentences pinned upon the board, exhibits labelled and words made with blocks and plastic letters, rather than by sitting still at a desk. The more practical use the child finds for the written word the greater the interest. The child's movements are at first big and bold. He can write on the blackboard and only much later can he learn to write on paper. It is also easier to make vertical movements on a board than horizontal ones on paper. This is why walls prove irresistible for early writing practice.

The child's ability to understand and use numbers tends to develop rather later than his understanding of written words. Although many children can count when they start school few have any real concept of numbers. Small children can think of numbers only in sequence. They can count fingers or beads and add one at a time, but they cannot think of numbers as entities or configurations. In a practical way, by using money, giving change, serving in the school shop, counting out bottles of milk or giving out books, the child learns to use numbers without acquiring a fear of arithmetic. The psychologist Piaget has shown that the number concept is very complex. The idea that number operations are reversible, for instance, is not really grasped until the child is about 7 or 8 years old (for example you can add 5 to any number and take it away again to arrive at the original number). The concept of number may entail the idea of size and an understanding of what to be bigger means. The figure 9 does not only come after 8 in counting, it is also bigger. Nine children are more than 8, 9 pennies are more than 8. Nine remains more than 8, whichever way the items are arranged. Small children have difficulty in understanding this. They may believe that 9 pennies laid on the table far apart are more money than 9 pennies in a small pile. The concept of number may involve the idea of classification and of manipulating 'sets'. Three boys and 4 girls, for example, are 7 children. The boys and girls are separate 'sets', children is a 'set' which includes both the other sets.

Small children can count and use the words for numbers, but, at first, the more complex understanding of number is beyond them. By about the age of 6 or 7 the child can sometimes carry out an arithmetical operation, at other times he appears completely unable to understand the problem. Piaget calls the phase of sporadic understanding 'intuitive thought'. In the next phase of the child's development he can solve problems in a practical way when he has objects which he can count and arrange. Piaget calls this the stage of 'concrete operational thought'. Only later can he perform the same test without the actual manipulation of objects. Piaget calls this the level of 'formal operational thought'. These phases of thought development—intuitive, concrete operational and formal operational—with transitional phases in which the child sometimes operates on a concrete and sometimes on a formal level, apply not only to his grasp of number but to all his intellectual activities. Successful schooling is achieved if teaching is adapted to the child's level of development.

The method of teaching which allows each child to progress at his own speed, to develop interests and to learn by doing rather than by sitting still is often referred to as the 'free activity method'. This term is often misunderstood by parents, who think that their children are not taught anything at all, and also by those who confuse free activity with bad behaviour. Where free activity methods are used behaviour is, as a rule, no worse—if not better—than in a more formal classroom. Moving about, talking and handling equipment are approved of where free activity is the method of choice. These activities are natural to a child and can be suppressed only by methods which may create fear and are therefore not conducive to learning. 'Open plan' schools without formal classrooms exploit fully the child's ability to learn while doing; visitors are often surprised at the hive of industry and lack of noise.

Discipline

Most children want to conform. They do not always know what is expected of them and have to be told, or they may know but have forgotten. However, they only need to be reminded and will immediately correct their behaviour. The process of socialisation is already well advanced by the time the child enters school. The parents' methods of exercising control are well understood; but the same rules may not necessarily apply at the school and the child has to experiment with the extent to which it will comply with the demands of teachers and peer group.

Sometimes it is great fun for them to be difficult and to see just how far it is possible to go in order to establish a right to be contrary. All children play this game at some time; and in every class, with every teacher, it must be played at least once. This is a way of getting to know the teacher, leading to a very clear understanding of the teacher's personality. Each teacher acquires a reputation of sternness or leniency, of being just or erratic, of being bad-tempered or placid as the result of the manner in which he deals with those children who try him out. It does not much matter how soon he draws the limits or what methods he uses, his peculiarities will become known and the class will settle down to a particular pattern of accepted behaviour. When the class has settled down, however, bad behaviour must be taken seriously because it may be an indication of more deep-rooted trouble. Persistent bad behaviour may be the only way in which some children succeed in gaining recognition. They may be so discouraged that they no longer try to do good work or to impress by their good behaviour. To be noticed at all they must be bad.

Some children may have failed to establish sufficiently satisfactory relationships with the teacher to want to please. Some may find that they can gain esteem among other children only by being a hero in taking punishment. When a child's behaviour is persistently out of step with the others punishment cannot really help and one must try to understand the underlying cause. This does not mean that punishment is necessarily wrong. Good teachers do not need to resort to physical punishment, but their reprimand or other forms of punishment can be more hurtful than corporal punishment.

The child's growing awareness of right and wrong carries with it the belief that a choice can be made between the right and the wrong act. Freedom of choice to behave badly gives the wrongdoer the right to be punished. We punish only when we think the child could have acted in a different way. If we do not think that he could have chosen any other action we absolve him from blame. A child who deliberately chooses to act wrongly may be asking to be punished and it may be necessary to respond to his demand. He may, in fact, feel guilty about something unknown to the teacher and his subsequent naughtiness may be a device for getting punished for two things at once. Or he may be trying to confirm in his own mind his judgment about right or wrong. If, for example, he thinks he is doing the wrong thing by arriving late and yet nobody takes it seriously he becomes confused about his own standards and he has to try again until eventually he is punished.

Inconsistency by the teacher may lead to bad behaviour which could have been avoided without much punishment. Small children like to conform. They feel secure when there are firm limits to their behaviour. They enjoy the approval of the adult. Later they accept adult standards as their own and self-discipline can be encouraged. Inconsistency in parents and teachers early in the child's life leads to confusion of standards.

Learning, Intelligence

Progress during school years depends, among other factors, on the child's intelligence and on his motivation for learning.

It is well known to teachers that in spite of all efforts children learn at different rates. The French psychologist Binet was one of the first to attempt to determine whether ability to learn is innate or whether methods of education can affect the child's progress. He tried to choose questions and tests which were, as far as possible, independent of the educational achievements of the children he tested. He selected tests for the youngest age groups in such a way that a child with normal physique and normal opportunities could not fail to learn the required responses. Such skills as tying up laces, copying a square, cutting paper, stringing beads according to a given pattern are among the test items. For older children there are pictures in which some essential part is missing, questions about the correct thing to do in common circumstances. For very much older children or adults some of the test items require the ability to read, but apart from this, educational achievement is not tested.

Items for the test were finally selected in such a manner that when 50 per cent of the children of any given age successfully completed them they were considered to measure the normal intelligence of that age group. Children who only completed tests for a younger age group were considered to have the 'mental age' of a younger child. Those who succeeded in tests beyond their age had a higher mental than chronological age. The comparison of chronological and mental age, calculated as follows, was called the intelligence quotient.

$$\frac{\text{Mental Age}}{\text{Chronological Age}} \times 100 = \text{Intelligence Quotient}$$

When mental age and chronological age are the same the intelligence quotient is 100.

Since Binet's tests were first published many others have appeared; some are easier to administer, some are more suitable for adults or for more intelligent people than Binet's test is able to assess, but basically the principles of intelligence measurement are those which Binet devised.

Binet discovered among the children he tested that the relationship between mental age and chronological age remained fairly constant however often he tested the children; the intelligence quotient was apparently innate. We now realise that innate intelligence cannot really be measured and that intelligence tests can only measure the performance of which the child is capable, partly as a result of his innate ability and partly as a result of the influence of his environment. Increasingly we have become aware of the need for an encouraging, stimulating environment, early in life, to enable the child to make full use of his innate intelligence. There are some children so deprived of opportunities to develop that they appear to be of very low intelligence. After a change to a more stimulating environment, for example a move from an institution to a foster home, the increase in the score on intelligence tests can be quite dramatic.

We know that intelligence tests measure something which is closely related to the ability to learn. Spearman, an English psychologist, described intelligence as consisting of several factors, one, which he called 'g', representing a general overall ability to learn. The others, which he called 's', are specific factors, enabling people to learn one special subject, for example, music or geometry or languages, more easily than other subjects. Tests differ in the extent to which they are able to measure 'g' or 's'.

Children with high intelligence usually have high 'g'; they are generally more able to profit from teaching and are good at most subjects. Contrary to popular belief many intelligent children are good at school subjects as well as sports, arts and practical subjects such as cooking and sewing. They may develop special interests or receive more encouragement in some of their activities than in others, but high intelligence would enable them to be more successful than less intelligent children in whatever subject they chose to study. Intelligence remains fairly constant throughout life. Good assessment even at a fairly early age could give a reasonably reliable indication of a child's chances at school.

There are, however, few reliable tests and the administration of tests to small children is so difficult that most people feel doubtful about test results before the age of about 11 years. If the child is unwell, or in a bad mood, results may underestimate the child's intelligence. Children develop very rapidly during the first few school years, there are sometimes sudden bursts of developing insight into the kind of problems which intelligence tests present. Increased interest in the child's progress at home and changes in home environment may increase test scores considerably over a period of one or two years; however, practice or coaching in the use of intelligence tests produces only a very small amount of improvement.

High scores in intelligence tests can almost certainly be accepted as a measurement of high ability. Low scores may underestimate the child. Intelligence is normally distributed in the population. This means that nearly 70 per cent of all people have an intelligence quotient of or near 100. Fifteen per cent are more intelligent and 15 per cent less intelligent. The top 5 to 10 per cent are of outstanding ability, often referred to as 'genius'. The lowest 3 to 5 per cent of all children have such low intelligence that they require special care throughout life. Binet's findings have influenced educational practice in most countries.

We believe that all children should be educated according to their ability. There are special schools or classes for those whose slowness in learning requires special methods of teaching. Many people believe that the brightest, too, may need special schools if their interest in learning is to be maintained. There is some controversy about the education of the largest group of children whose intelligence deviates only a little from the average. Teaching is easiest if children in one class are evenly matched in intelligence, but some authorities prefer to encourage children of varying ability to learn together.

In order to learn effectively there must be adequate motivation. In infant schools and among university students the subjects are of such intrinsic interest that learning carries its own reward. The most powerful incentives are success and approval. Punishment, criticism, ridicule can act as incentives for only a very short time. Encouragement, praise, rewards and success stimulate learning indefinitely. Those who favour streaming in schools believe success comes more easily to children in such classes. It is bad for the child to remain constantly at the bottom of the class and to be doomed to failure in competition. Those who feel less favourable to streaming believe that each child's success should be measured in relation to its own previous performance and that it is wrong to encourage children to compete with each other, that it is possible to teach children without encouraging competition.

Controversy about selection reaches its climax when children move from primary to secondary schools. The Education Act of 1944 provided different types of schools for children of different ability. It was suggested that the school most suited to each child's ability should be selected. Grammar schools were to be chosen for those children whose ability appeared to make them suitable for education leading towards university entrance. Technical and secondary modern schools were to cater for the rest of them.

The subject matter taught in grammar schools and their methods of teaching were to be adapted to the ability of the most able pupils and selection procedures were devised to find those children most likely to benefit from the course of study offered in these schools.

Secondary modern schools and technical schools were to be able to adapt their syllabus and teaching methods to the interest and ability of the other pupils so that each pupil could obtain the education best suited to him. This system did not work entirely satisfactorily. Many parents have not really believed that the best type of school had been selected for their child. They interpreted the selection procedure as one in which the child was submitted to a selection test which he had to pass in order to get into a grammar school. Those who did not obtain a place in a grammar school often experienced this as a failure and secondary modern schools were regarded by many people as inferior. Comprehensive schools, where children of all ranges of ability are educated together, have now largely replaced the former divisive system of schooling.

Selection of a secondary modern school was intended to ensure that the child should not suffer from failure in competition with brighter children if all were to be educated together.

In effect, failure to reach grammar school was interpreted by many as failure in competition and therefore secondary modern schools did not succeed in giving children of average ability sufficient motivation for learning.

Many people now prefer not to rely on intelligence tests at any particular age and to encourage all children to progress according to their ability and rate of maturation. Recent evidence from junior schools has shown that the general level of attainment is sometimes higher in unstreamed than in streamed schools. As an example of this we could take two children with the same reading score who enter a junior school at the age of 7 years. One is placed in the A stream and soon finds herself bottom of the class while the other is doing very well in the B stream. Two years later both children are again tested but in spite of her discouraging experience the child in the A stream is found to be better in reading ability than her friend in the B stream. The fact that she had been placed in the A stream had proved to be a better incentive than being top of the class. (Other researchers have, however, shown that initial failure in academic work has resulted in progressive retardation owing to the emotional trauma set up. This applies particularly to adolescents and adults.)

Whatever the form of selection for secondary schooling it is essential that encouragement and optimism should prevail both at home and in school and that the child should steadily widen his interest, knowledge and skill in order that he may approach adulthood with confidence.

SUGGESTIONS FOR FURTHER READING

DANZIGER, K. *Socialization*. Harmondsworth: Penguin, 1971.

ERIKSON, E. H. *Childhood and Society*. Revised ed. Harmondsworth: Pelican, 1965.

FRAIBERG, S. H. and M. *The Magic Years*. New York: Scribner's, 1959; London. Methuen, 1968.

GESELL, A. *et al. The First Five Years of Life*. London: Methuen, 1955.

ISAACS, S. *Intellectual Growth in Young Children*. London: Routledge, 1930.

ISAACS, S. *Social Development in Young Children*. London: Routledge, 1933.

JACKSON, B. *Streaming: An Education System in Miniature*. London: Routledge, 1964.

LORENZ, K. Z. *King Solomon's Ring*. London: Methuen (University Paperbacks), 1961.

MILLAR, S. *The Psychology of Play*. Harmondsworth: Penguin, 1968.

NEWSON, J. and NEWSON, E. *Infant Care in an Urban Community*. Harmondsworth: Penguin, 1963.

NEWSON, J. and NEWSON, E. *Four Years Old in an Urban Community*. Harmondsworth: Penguin, 1969.

PIAGET, J. *The Language and Thought of the Child*, 3rd ed. revised. London: Routledge, 1959.

SCHAFFER, H. R. *The Growth of Sociability*. Harmondsworth: Penguin, 1971.

STEVENSON, H. C. *Child Psychology*. Chicago: University of Chicago Press, 1963.

VALENTINE, C. W. *The Normal Child and some of his Abnormalities*. Harmondsworth: Penguin, 1956.

WINNICOTT, D. W. *The Child, the Family and the Outside World*. Harmondsworth: Penguin, 1964.

5. ADOLESCENCE

There is no precise definition of adolescence. Adults refer to adolescence as the age in which young people are no longer children but are not yet grown up. Children, looking to the future, do not contemplate adolescence, only adulthood. Adolescents may not recognise themselves as such, preferring to be known by some other term, such as 'teenager'. Growing up is a gradual process involving physical, intellectual, emotional and social growth. Development in these various ways does not always occur smoothly. Around the age of 14 intelligence reaches its maximum and physical development may be very advanced or very much retarded. Emotional and social development are very incomplete.

The young person may find this period one of special difficulty, but there are many people whose secure early environment enables them to pass through adolescence without difficulty. The rapid development of intelligence may create conflict between parent and child. The adolescent, who is conscious of his intellectual superiority, may, at the same time, become aware of the occasional faulty judgment of his elders. He has not yet gained the necessary experience of life to apply his intelligence well, nor the maturity to make allowances for the older generation. He suddenly realises that his knowledge and power of reasoning are equal or superior to his parents' and becomes aware that parents, who hitherto had been thought of as paragons, can be fallible. The adolescent is still sufficiently childish to believe that if parents are wrong in one thing they must always be wrong; that if he himself is right in one thing he is always right. This attitude of absolute self-confidence in his own judgment is sometimes irritating to older people. When parents are in fact of lower intelligence than their children, or less well educated, they may strongly resent the intellectual superiority and the cocksure manner of their children and they may feel that their children are beyond their control. Adolescents delight in catching older people out and can be quite merciless to teachers or other adults once they have lost confidence in their judgment. On the other hand, they unreservedly admire those superior qualities which they most desire for themselves. Hero-worship is a characteristic of the adolescent stage.

Physical development is particularly erratic in adolescence. Sexual maturity may occur as early as 11 or 12 years and as late as 16 to 17 years. Physical growth occurs suddenly and unevenly. The proportion of feet and hands to limbs or limbs to trunk may change rapidly; facial growth may radically alter the appearance. The result is often seen in a physical awkwardness which makes life almost intolerably miserable. Unthinking adults may aggravate the situation by commenting on the adolescent's clumsiness, gawkiness or ungainly appearance. To a certain extent participation in sports can help to overcome physical awkwardness. Clothes become extremely important in making the adolescent feel comfortable. There is no greater humiliation than clothes which have become too tight or too short, or look too childish or too dowdy. Many adolescents, especially girls, feel so strongly about clothes that they prefer to leave school as soon as they can rather than wear school uniform, which they believe accentuates their physical disadvantages. The fact that adolescents feel unsure about their physical appearance often causes them to spend a considerable amount of time in front of the mirror in order to get used to their altered body image. Girls experiment with hair-styles and make-up, for example, and often worry a good deal about their figure. If their breasts have not yet developed they feel childish and conspicuous, yet when they do develop they worry about them becoming too big. They often worry about weight increase and experiment with slimming diets. Boys take some time to get used to their new voice when it has broken. They may feel ambivalent about their growth of beard and about the necessity to shave.

During adolescence, detachment from family ties occurs and independence is established. In the most favourable circumstances detachment from the home is gradual while interests widen, friendships are formed among people of the same age and adult models are found outside the family circle. Frequently, however, the period of detachment from home is stormy and disturbed.

Adolescents, who are still in the habit of making wild generalisations, of seeing issues in black and white, of wholehearted acceptance or rejection, may suddenly experience a most powerful rejection of all that their family stands for. They may go to opposite extremes from parental values in their views about religion, morals, or their future careers. They may fight their battles with parents on these important issues or they may do so on relatively unimportant matters, such as clothes, tastes in interior decoration, methods of spending their leisure or opinions about music.

Some adolescents find in religion the support they require. The search for absolute values, trust in God and the understanding of metaphysical concepts may be of immense value to them during this period of emotional insecurity. The ultimately accepted religious beliefs and ethical codes may not be those of the parents but rather those arrived at by the adolescent's own struggle for truth.

Most adolescents gain support in their struggle for independence from others of their own age. The approval and admiration of members of their own age group becomes much more important than the approval of adults. Adolescents need to form groups and to belong wholeheartedly to them. At school there is evidence of gang formation and complete conformity to the standards of the gang is essential. The word 'gang' may not denote undesirable group formation, but expresses the peculiar adolescent way of forming rival units distinctive in dress, in speech or in some other outward sign in such a way that members of the gang can recognise each other instantly and also members of rival groups. Each member of the group accepts and adopts unquestioningly the mannerisms, opinions, habits of the other members. Unless conformity is absolute there is no way of indicating loyalty to the group. Fashions in hair-styles, in clothes, in popular songs and in spare-time activities are created in this way by adolescents. The ethics of the gang are in marked contrast to the self-centred thinking of the small child. Whether the fashions are socially acceptable or not depends partly on the leadership and opportunities of the group, partly on the extent to which adults create antagonism in the adolescent. Even membership of a delinquent group is, from the point of view of the mental health of the adolescent, better than going through adolescence as an isolated individual, or remaining too closely attached to the family group.

Crazes about ballet, concerts and visits to art galleries are as much the manifestation of adolescent gregariousness as are dance halls and street-corner gatherings. The latter tend to evoke more criticism from adults and thereby may become more obviously antisocial. Youth clubs may sometimes satisfy adolescent needs for recognition. Some social organisations, the scout movement for example, deliberately attempt to satisfy the need for uniform and instant recognition of members. Badges, rituals, sign language all make it easier to identify members of the group. Very often, however, young people feel dissatisfied with the organisations of the scout kind because they are too formal. They like youth clubs organised by themselves, not for them. At the time of their greatest antagonism to adults they cannot tolerate adult patronage.

The adolescent's position in society is very ill-defined. Parents and teachers expect adult behaviour and attitudes, yet they are unwilling to treat the adolescent as an equal. He resents being treated as a child, yet he finds comfort at times in behaving like one. If the adolescent is still at school he feels inferior to those who until recently were his equals but who have entered the adult world of work and are earning money. Those who start working find that they are not really accepted as adults by the world in general. Youth, inexperience and lack of knowledge are constantly held against them reproachfully. In some primitive societies transition from childhood to adulthood is made easier by definite, prescribed 'initiation rites'. In our social structure adolescents belong to neither the adult nor childhood fraternity and the path to adulthood has to be found by trial and error.

It is difficult for children to have any clear conception of adulthood. The fact that adults have duties and obligations as well as rights is quite unknown even to adolescents. Their choice of work or careers may be based on completely unrealistic ideas and their first experiences of adult life are very disappointing. Adults are not only expected to accept responsibility willingly for their own actions, but sometimes, indeed, for the actions of others, a fact for which adolescents are often ill prepared.

It is sometimes difficult for the young person to deal with the change in status which accompanies changing roles in family, school and work. Within the family the child's status may increase as he begins to contribute financially and as he becomes independent. Outside the family the senior pupils of a school enjoy relatively high status in relation to the other pupils and even the teachers treat them with a certain amount of respect. To assume a position of low status at the place of work or in the junior ranks of an institute of higher education may be very painful to the adolescent's self-esteem.

Emotional as well as social development may reach an unstable point in adolescence. Children experience rapidly changing strong emotions and are able and allowed to express these freely and immediately in words or actions. Adults can control the expression of emotions and experience lasting rather than rapidly changing ones. Children react rapidly to people and things, showing strong liking or disliking of people and sometimes anger at objects which happen to be in their way. Adults differentiate in their emotional reaction to people —they love some very deeply but are emotionally unaffected by others. They may devote deep feeling to ideas such as patriotism, pacificism, justice. Children need to be loved and adults need to give love. The adolescent's emotions lie somewhere between those of childhood and adulthood. He feels deeply but often indiscriminately. He may not yet be able to control the expression of feelings yet, in trying to do so, he may give the impression of being cold and hard. He is beginning to feel strongly about ideas but covers his feeling with bumptiousness or the appearance of being opinionated. He still needs to be loved but cannot accept it without feeling self-conscious. He is beginning to give love, not yet for the satisfaction of other people's needs, but rather because he obtains emotional satisfaction from giving. At this particular moment of emotional turmoil the adolescent may become aware, perhaps for the first time, of sexual urges and desires. He may be unsure of the way to deal with his sexual feelings and unable to discuss them. In the next pages we shall refer again to sexual development and to the help which may be needed in the form of sex education. Sexual feelings are mentioned here only as yet another difficulty in the adolescent's experience of life.

Some young people indulge, for a time, in behaviour which adults regard as delinquent. There may be a number of reasons for this. Some behaviour, for example, which, a few years earlier, would merely have been regarded as naughty, becomes delinquent in adolescents mainly because adolescents, by virtue of their greater strength and size, can be so much more destructive. Throwing stones, for example, is an innocent pastime with some nuisance value when a child is small, but it becomes vandalism in adolescence. Fights among small boys are relatively harmless, among adolescents there can be serious injury.

Some delinquent behaviour occurs almost accidentally because of the young people's tendency to form gangs. Some adolescents live in such cramped, uninteresting surroundings that almost any activity results in annoyance to someone near by. The provision of sports centres and playing fields and facilities for getting into the country, to the mountains or the sea, may help young people who find themselves frustrated by lack of space. Some housing estates are particularly unsuited to the interests of adolescents. Having originally been built for young couples with small children they have failed to develop a real community feeling. In the absence of meeting places, dance halls, cinemas or any other community centres young people are obliged to meet in the street or in cafés and often find insufficient outlet for their energies. One of the additional problems of housing estates arises from the fact that the age distribution of the population is quite unlike that of older communities. Having, in the first instance, been provided for young couples and small children they are now populated by middle-aged adults and adolescents. There are few old people, few young adults and few small children. The young people, who are now adolescent, have grown up without any models of older children to copy and without their guidance into adolescence.

While it is true that delinquency occurs chiefly among adolescents, less among adults, it is not true to say that most adolescents are delinquent. It is only when adolescents are antisocial, even in relation to their own peers, or when they have grown to distrust all people and to hate all authority, that their delinquencies give cause for concern. Some young people have the desire to enlarge their experience by experimenting with drugs. While sensational newspaper articles have probably exaggerated the problem there is justifiable cause for alarm. It is particularly worrying that adolescents are easy prey for drug pedlars, who earn their living by introducing new customers to the use of drugs and who, by bringing young drug takers into contact with the underworld, can easily lead them on to more serious forms of delinquency. Many young people have sufficient stability and common sense to give up drugs after experimentation, having realised that it is simply not worth it. Others need education and information about the dangers of the first steps on the road to drug addiction and they need protection from those who try to involve them in this kind of behaviour.

With so many problems reaching their climax in adolescence it is surprising how successfully most children pass on to adulthood. Recognition by adults of all that is good and positive in young people contributes perhaps more than anything else to the self-confidence necessary in adolescence.

Sexual Development

During adolescence physical development reaches its maturity. Changes in glandular functions, in physique, voice and facial expression, may increase the adolescent's self-consciousness and emotional turmoil. With the awareness of bodily readiness the adolescent may experience sexual urges and emotional changes which may be frightening and profoundly disturbing. The climax of sexual development is reached later, in adulthood, when bodily maturation is accompanied by the ability to love and to choose a partner with

whom a permanent relationship of marriage and the foundation of family life are wholly satisfactory. Adult sexuality
consists not only of the unique relationship between one man
and one woman which makes intercourse a profoundly
satisfying experience to both, but also of being able to love
the partner to the exclusion of all others. To enter into a
permanently binding relationship entails a complete reorientation of attitudes, interest and social adjustment, changes
which make it possible later to enter into parenthood and to
give children the love and affection they need. Physical
relationship without an accompanying emotional development cannot be considered complete. Sexual urges and sexual
behaviour do not suddenly manifest themselves in adolescents,
but adolescent and adult sexual behaviour are stages of a
gradual development which begins at birth.

For a long period during the early school years the child is
entirely engaged in social learning. Not until he reaches early
adolescence is his interest in his body reawakened. The young
adolescent has sufficient factual knowledge to associate his
genital organs with sex, he is aware of his bodily tensions and
recognises them as being sexual. One method of relieving
sexual tension is masturbation. Nearly everyone masturbates
at some time in their lives. Kinsey, in his investigations in the
U.S.A., put the incidence as high as 92 per cent for men and
nearly 60 per cent for women. It is the belief in some religions
that masturbation is sinful and many young people feel intensely guilty about their indulgence. For this reason they keep
their practice strictly secret. They believe that they alone are
guilty of such practices and their guilt feeling increases corre-
spondingly. Some people also believe, erroneously, that
masturbation is harmful. The conviction in medical quarters
is that masturbation is not the cause of any psychotic disorders.
Most people abandon the practice for other sexual activity
when a suitable sexual partner is available. The adolescent

does not always, however, have this information available. His parents may still disapprove of the practice, or condemn it, or the adolescent may think they do and he may refrain from confiding in them. He may have developed sufficient inhibitions to make it difficult for him to obtain sexual information from his parents or to discuss sexual problems with them. This becomes even more marked in the next phase when emotionally he becomes interested in people of his own sex. This homosexual phase in development is normal and needs to be understood as such by the adolescent so that he can see it as a temporary phase leading to adult heterosexual interest.

Quite suddenly the adolescent may become interested in the opposite sex. For a long period boys and girls consider each other to be stupid and friendships, therefore, are made almost entirely with their own sex. At that stage there is little concern for appearance. Those, for instance, who are interested in clothes or cosmetics are ridiculed. Suddenly interest in the other sex is aroused or rather the adolescent seeks to awaken the interest of the opposite sex. Emotionally the need is still to be loved and noticed rather than to give love. Girls begin to take care of their clothes, hair and personal hygiene, become interested in fashion and seek advice about beauty in women's magazines. Boys smarten up in appearance and both sexes give up childhood's games and interests. This phase strikes adults as being the awakening of sexual urges. In fact it should be seen to be only one phase though at times it may be a particularly stormy one.

The adolescent is still groping for standards of beauty and moral behaviour. He is conscious of his looks but does not know if his looks appeal to the opposite sex. Attempts at choosing clothes, using cosmetics, selecting jewellery often meet with derision from adults instead of evoking encouragement and offers of help. The result often is that parental standards are deliberately rejected. Adolescents find each other attractive because of the obvious effort each makes despite the fact that there may be little that could be called aesthetic success.

Adolescents usually want to do the right and proper thing, but they find it difficult to discover what is right. They give up playing childish games and pursuing childish interests because these seem obviously out of place, yet they have nothing to substitute so they spend hours doing nothing at all. Adults are bored and irritated by this refusal to develop interests and it gives rise to friction in the home and to deterioration in school work, sometimes at the age at which effort at school may be most desirable. Many people are worried about the apparent waste of time which occurs during the last year in secondary modern schools, but forget the need for a period during which boys and girls may discover what is likely to be expected of them when they have grown up.

Boys sometimes find the transition to manhood easier than girls find transition to womanhood. Girls, who are less free to experiment with methods of self-expression and self-display, may not find their feminine role easily identifiable. Adjustment to work, on the other hand, is more easily accomplished by girls than by boys.

General interest in the opposite sex usually gives way to a specific interest in one person of the opposite sex. While there is general interest mixed social gatherings in dance halls, clubs or coffee bars are attended and enjoyed. Couple formation disrupts social gatherings. The two people concerned are interested only in each other, so they usually leave the group and find enjoyment where they can be alone. Most youth clubs suffer constant depletion from among their senior and more reliable members and, because of this, come to rely on adult leadership. There may be many rapid changes in the attraction felt towards a person of the opposite sex. Dating and flirtations are necessary experiences before the right person for marriage can be found. At this stage the adolescent is learning to give love as well as to receive it. It may be given profusely and gushingly and often may be unacceptar to the other. The emotion of love often overflows and embraces society as a whole; there is an overwhelming desire to do good, to be of service, to care for others.

By the time sexually mature relationship is possible love is given to satisfy the needs of others rather than purely selfish needs. Interests become adapted to those of others, opinions change in accordance with others and activities cease to be self-centred.

Adult sexual and emotional relationships are completely satisfying. Some people believe that this is so to such an extent that there is little energy left for activities of social usefulness. They believe that wholehearted devotion to the arts, or science or business, or the care of other people's children is possible only as a substitute for sexual satisfaction. The term 'sublimation' is used to describe this feeling for some cause which is entirely satisfying and not consciously connected with sexual satisfaction. Many people, however, if they fail to find sexual satisfaction, retain a longing which they are unable to admit even to themselves and which leaves them angry and dissatisfied.

In order to lead a full, normal life each stage of development must give rise to satisfaction. This does not mean that people should be encouraged to give way to all sexual urges and impulses. It means that in the early stages the child's need for love and food must be satisfied. Later he must learn to recognise his feelings and deal with them consciously. If guilt feelings are associated with sexual thoughts this makes it impossible to talk about and control difficulties. Instruction in sexual development is essential in order to avoid the confusion in standards which results from guilt feelings and secrecy. Most parents believe that the best way of teaching their children about sex is simply to answer all questions frankly and simply when they arise. It must be remembered, however, that children's questions may not fully reflect their misconceptions and they may ask questions so badly that the parents' answer becomes irrelevant. Even simple answers can be very bewildering. Children may, for example, know that babies grow inside the mother's abdomen. What they are puzzled about may be how the seed got in or how the baby comes out. Some children feel sure that the seed must be eaten to get in and, because they often think they too could have babies if they tried, they may develop food fads or abnormal preoccupations about food in the fear of becoming pregnant. Children may believe that kissing is the way to start a baby and may, for a time, become reluctant to kiss anyone. The umbilicus is sometimes thought to be the place through which babies are born and fears of the abdomen splitting open occur. Other children believe that bowel or bladder functions are associated with childbirth.

Some of the irrational beliefs of young children still exist in adolescents or are reactivated. Many young people reach adolescence without full knowledge of biological facts, or secretly afraid that they are not fully informed. Many moral problems may trouble the adolescent and he needs an opportunity for full and free discussion of sexual matters.

Parents inevitably have anxious moments and thoughts about the sexual problems of their children. The solution of this dilemma does not consist of warnings against possible dangers before the true significance of sex is understood, but in building up over the years a relationship of confidence, trust and understanding. Frankness is essential but tact and understanding are also necessary. Sometimes it is better for a person outside the family to advise the adolescent on matters of sex. Emotional reactions may be quite strong even in families which pride themselves on their open frankness on most topics.

SUGGESTIONS FOR FURTHER READING

FLEMING, C. M. *Adolescence*. 2nd ed. revised. London: Routledge, 1967.

HAVIGHURST, R. J. and TABA, H. *Adolescent Character and Personality*. New York: Wiley, 1949.

MILLER, D. *Growth to Freedom*. London: Tavistock, 1968.

NEWELL, P. *et al*. *Teenagers and Drugs*. An Education Pamphlet, 1966.

ODLUM, D. M. *Journey through Adolescence*. Revised and enlarged ed. London: Delisle, 1965.

RAISON, T. *Youth in New Society*. London: Hart-Davis, 1966.

6. MATURITY

Children and adolescents look forward to adulthood. Yet when this is reached it may still be felt that something is lacking. The sense of satisfaction, of completeness, which for so long has been anticipated, is not experienced and they still feel that there must be some way in which the purpose of maturity can be more adequately fulfilled. 'Maturity' is spoken of as being the highest aim. Because most people aim higher than their current achievement maturity is elusive, always to be aimed at, never to be reached. The more mature an individual's behaviour is the more it is likely that he is aware of those qualities within himself which are still undeveloped and doubt is often expressed as to whether anyone can ever be said to be mature, or whether any definition is entirely adequate.

It may be easier to speak of 'integration of personality' rather than of maturity, because the concept of 'maturing', which means 'ripening', implies that an optimal stage may be reached and that later a decline sets in. This is true of 'intelligence' which reaches optimal values in adolescence and declines from the middle thirties onwards. Integration of the various aspects of personality, however, may continue throughout life.

Emotional Growth

Since it is difficult to describe a mature person it may be helpful to consider trends in development which lead towards desirable stages of adulthood and to examine the ideals which should be kept in mind when maturity is sought. The most important changes taking place during growth lie in the range of emotional experiences and the manner in which emotions find expression. Infants react to a very small number of stimuli; adults to a very large number. Infants have a very limited selection of emotional responses; adults have a large range of emotions. Infants react with immediate response; adults can delay and control emotional expression. In childhood emotion is aroused equally by objects, people and events. As the individual gets older emotional response is increasingly evoked by abstract concepts and ideas. Infants and small children react irresponsibly; adults take responsibility not only for their own actions but also for those of their subordinates.

Emotional maturity, then, entails the ability to withhold or delay emotional responses and to display and express emotion in a socially accepted manner. Temper tantrums, for example, are disapproved of in most societies, but grief or pleasure may be freely displayed in some cultures. British people by reason of training show a minimum of emotional display. It is, however, necessary to retain the ability to feel emotions deeply, strongly and lastingly. To do this people must learn to recognise their emotions and not to deny that they exist. While it is wise to help children to control their behaviour it is dangerous to make them feel guilty about their feelings. If the strength of a child's emotion becomes too frightening he grows up as if he had never had the emotional experience and emotion becomes unconscious and inaccessible. Many adults are motivated in their behaviour by emotions which properly belong to childhood, but which have never been adequately dealt with because they were too rapidly pushed into unconsciousness. It is a part of maturity to recognise that actions are not always entirely rational. A large area of personality is unconscious and much of what appears to be well-reasoned behaviour results from unconscious emotional motivation.

The objects of emotion change during the maturing process. Inanimate things no longer arouse feelings; instead the individual feels strongly about people. In childhood the mother, later the father, and then relatives and friends matter a great deal. There is a great need to be loved. All emotion is self-centred. All new knowledge is evaluated according to the child's own feelings about it. People are seen as good or bad according to the way they impinge on his emotions.

The adolescent is still preoccupied with his own feelings and is critical of others because they do not sufficiently satisfy his emotional needs. However, he experiences a change from the need to be loved by his parents to a need for acceptance by a community of peers. The feeling of belonging to a group becomes most important and with this he develops the ability to assess how others feel, what others expect, what pleases them and to assess, to some extent, how others will react to his own behaviour.

During adolescence there is increasing need to give rather than to receive. At first this is all-embracing. The adolescent feels strongly for all the members of his group. He obtains satisfaction from giving and searches for people on whom he can bestow his love. Children, animals, helpless people, become the object of his emotional bounty. Soon he becomes more selective and seeks reciprocity for his emotion until, in marriage, there is complete satisfaction in the love given to and received from his partner.

Parenthood entails a change in emotion towards an entirely altruistic attitude of giving love. Possessive mothers love their children because they need to be loved in return and because they derive satisfaction from being able to give. Completely mature motherhood would make it possible to give all the love the child needs without taking anything in return and for the child's sake entirely, not for the mother's own satis-faction. It is difficult to say whether this completely unselfish love is ever possible. Whenever the question arises whether an unloved or orphaned child should be adopted or placed in a foster home one must try to find out how far the prospective mother is able to satisfy a child's needs and to what extent her desire to take in a child is a result of her own need to be loved by a child. There is a great danger that children who were deprived of love early in life may take a long time before they can respond to mothering. If the motive for taking in the child is not entirely altruistic the mother, disappointed by a lack of response from the child, may reject him, regret her decision and blame the child for the failure.

In mature years it is possible to widen the scope for emotion and feel strongly about ideas and causes as well as about people. The psychologist Shand called this 'sentiment' and spoke, for example, of the sentiment of patriotism or of pacificism. A sentiment comprises all the emotions which may be felt in relation to a particular idea. Patriotism, for example, evokes pleasurable feelings when the country does well in competition; fear if it is threatened; anger if it is attacked. Perhaps the most mature people have the greatest number of sentiments and the widest range of interest. They have formed sentiments attached to more abstract ideas. This concern for events beyond the individual's own experience might be called a philosophy of life. The ability to become interested in people and ideas far removed from daily experience is closely related to one other aspect of maturity; namely, integration in society.

Social Growth

In our particular society adults have formed a fairly characteristic pattern of social grouping around themselves. They have a very close emotional bond with one other person, a bond different from any other relationship in its intensity and in the extent to which it is reciprocated. The relationship between husband and wife, or between mother and baby, are examples. A little further removed but still very close is a circle of a few people very important to one another; for example, the rest of the family and a set of close friends where the relationships are reciprocated. Any disaster occurring to any person in the circle would greatly affect every other person in it. This circle is formed during childhood, adolescence and early adulthood and does not change much after that. As people grow older it becomes progressively more difficult to admit new people into this very close relationship and, of course, the loneliness of old age is a result of the gradual thinning out of this circle. Within it, emotional bonds are so strong that they survive differences of opinion and separation in space and time.

A little further distant is a more populated circle of good friends, workmates and well-liked relations. These are people about whose welfare the individual still cares very much but whose disappearance causes him less concern. They have friends who are not included in one's own circle of friends. Behaviour towards this group of people is governed by social convention and learnt with difficulty during childhood. We can all think of examples of children's failure to distinguish the appropriate behaviour towards friends of their parents or even towards total strangers.

Apart from these closer relationships there are many people with whom the individual has some kind of social contact in a more and more distant way: the people with whom correspondence is maintained, people with whom Christmas cards are exchanged, people met on the way to work, tradesmen, bus conductors. Adults know how to behave towards all these people but think about them only during actual social contact. There is no reciprocity in relationship. The relationship between customer and salesman, for example, is totally different for each of the two people involved.

Maturity can, to some extent, be measured by the extent to which a person cares about the people in the distant circles of his social field and by finding out how far his social field extends. Children do not care about anyone they do not know personally. Adults begin to care about people in their street, or village, or club, even if they do not know them personally. An accident, or a case of cruelty to children, or poverty matters if it has happened to a friend. As maturity is reached such occurrences matter even if they happen in some other part of the country or in a foreign land. The sense of personal involvement in all that happens to human beings anywhere is again an expression of a philosophy of life.

Mature Attitude to Work

One other aspect of maturity will receive only brief mention in this chapter as it is more fully dealt with later. This is the mature person's attitude to work.

Late in adolescence or early in adulthood, a decision is made about work or choice of career. The way people decide on the work they wish to do is usually complex. Family influence, teachers' opinions, the glamour of propaganda, all enter into the choice of work but rarely succeed in the long run in deciding what is to be the individual's working life. Most people find it difficult to state what caused them to make their choice. The truth is that many factors enter into it, most of them unconscious.

Work is a contribution towards the well-being of society. Most people find it necessary to work because only in that way can they justify their existence. Many people say they work only for money, but, in fact, to be out of work even if there is no shortage of money is extremely demoralising. Disabled people, old people, and those without work during slumps have expressed their feeling of uselessness and their loss of self-respect during periods of idleness. Some people gain satisfaction from being useful to their family rather than from a contribution to society in general. Women often gain sufficient satisfaction from their usefulness to husband and children and feel that they do not need other work. Their work, however, is carried out in the home and may be all the more rewarding for being unpaid. The extent to which the work is seen to be useful gives it a certain amount of prestige. Many people gain satisfaction from their work because of the status it confers upon them. Anyone who feels that his work lacks prestige must either change his job or convince others of the importance of what he is doing.

The mature person may be one who has found satisfaction in his work and whose personal plans and ambitions have either found fulfilment or been submerged in a concern for the general well-being of the community. He is looking forwards and backwards at the same time, plans for the future are related to past achievements. Plans for the future are realistic and the ambitions and ideas of others are taken into account.

7. OLD AGE

Just as it is difficult to define adolescence and maturity, so also old age defies definition.

To children parents in the thirties appear old; grandparents seem ancient. As the years advance old age recedes and some people of 70 and 80 years do not consider themselves old at all. Maturity in social and emotional development may not occur until late in life and by that time the body may begin to lose its efficiency and intelligence may be declining. Damage to the brain tissue, owing to lack of oxygen, brain injury or infection may cause premature and exaggerated manifestations of ageing which are in no way characteristic of the ageing process of normal people.

Most people feel that they are getting old when they are physically unable to do all the things they still feel inclined to do. With advancing years breathlessness supervenes more easily, tiredness may be felt in the middle of the day. The older woman finds increasing difficulty in carrying out the chores at home in a reasonable time. This is often upsetting to her husband who may have retired but finds the house less relaxing than he had anticipated.

Gradually eyesight and possibly hearing becomes less acute. It is easier to become aware of failing eyesight. Often the onset of deafness is not perceived and many old people complain of other people's lack of consideration in not speaking clearly, not realising that the fault lies in their own deafness. It is even possible for them to become suspicious when people are laughing and to create hostility in others by their inability to hear. The suggestion that hearing aids might be used is often vigorously rejected, partly because the realisation of a disability is too painful, partly because old people are embarrassed by wearing these aids and also, after trying to use one, are bothered by the very strange noises they experience. When we hear well we succeed in picking out voices and speech from the general background noise and ignore the rest. As deafness advances more and more noises become inaudible. Hearing aids magnify all sounds and after a period of silence the irrelevant noises may become unbearable.

With increasing age the daily activities of washing, combing hair, pulling on stockings, become more and more strenuous. These activities, which during adult life are habitual and therefore accomplished without thought, become important activities occupying conscious thought.

It may become more difficult to remember what is happening although gross memory defect for recent events occurs only in the dementia of old age. However, the elderly person finds it more difficult to attend to many things at the same time and consequently fails to take in some information which may later be required, appearing then to have forgotten the information, but in reality never having grasped it. It happens often, on the other hand, that the apparent forgetfulness of the aged in fact represents refusal to accept information, especially if it is not in accordance with their accepted ideas. Contrary to the belief often held by old people themselves learning new material is perfectly possible in old age, though it may take a little longer. In normal senescence intelligence does not decline very markedly. Vocabulary remains at a high level, but, in intelligence tests the ability to solve certain problems in a given time diminishes. Incidental learning diminishes. The older a person is the more he only learns what he sets out to learn and the less does he pick up incidental information which he interprets as unrelated. The range of performance can be increased if the old person does not resist.

Some old people tend to think of everyone younger than themselves as children, just as children consider everyone else to be old. This attitude of old people leads to a certain amount of selfishness, condescension and what may appear to be interference in the life of younger people. In homes where grandparents, parents and children live together relations are sometimes strained by the fact that the grandparents treat the parents as if they were children.

On the other hand old people and young children usually get on extremely well as their relationship is quite natural, uncritical and accepting. Parents often feel that grandparents spoil small children, but there is no reason to believe that the genuine love and understanding which passes between alternate generations is in any way harmful.

Old people's habits are fairly well fixed, an asset when conscious efforts become difficult. Interference by younger people is quite understandably resented. The problems which must be resolved by the aged are related to their increasing loneliness as their contemporaries die, one by one, to the realisation that they must retire from work and accept the fact that they are no longer needed, and to the need to think about death and to come to terms with this thought.

We live in an adult-centred society which thinks most highly of the productive section of the community. According to our society the purpose of childhood is to get over it as fast as possible, and we talk of the problem of 'old age' as if old people served no purpose and were merely a burden. This is not the case in all societies. There are people who consider that childhood is of supreme value and that the function of adults is primarily to support the young. In some eastern societies old age is the period of life most cherished and esteemed and the time looked forward to throughout life.

If we are to solve our problem of old age we must try to stop looking at people as valuable only as long as they can work and put greater value on the fund of knowledge and experience old people have to offer.

The personal loneliness of the very old cannot be avoided, but the feelings of isolation can be overcome by widening as early as possible the circle of friends and acquaintances and by developing a sense of responsibility for the welfare of others. There is ample scope in voluntary work in local government or other local organisations for those who are still interested in others and free from personal obligations.

Retirement can be very traumatic, especially if too many years have been spent in the same job and too much interest has been given to work to the exclusion of outside interests.

The problem of when to retire is often discussed. Some people believe that work should be continued as long as possible. This may, however, lead to many difficulties, including the uncomfortable awareness of blocking promotion for younger, perhaps abler people. Old people's methods cannot be readily changed and although their own work may still reach a very high standard their rigidity may have adverse effects on the efficiency and morale of the people with whom they are working. If retirement is left entirely to the decision of the individual he may reach a stage at which he is no longer capable of recognising his limitations. Most damaging, however, is the fact that late retirement makes it impossible to take up new interests and there is a good deal to be said for early compulsory retirement when the individual is still young enough to start making new friends and taking up new interests.

In preparing for old age it seems wise to have so many interests and friends that life is still full even when some activities have to be given up. Much is being done by education authorities and much more could be done to encourage hobby activities for older people. Too many are restricted to gardening and knitting for their hobbies. Sewing, craft and cookery classes are held for older people in some areas. Townswomen's Guilds and social clubs for the aged often provide valuable meeting places and interesting activities, but encouragement and participation by younger people is necessary to ensure success. Some recent housing developments make it possible for the aged to live near their families as used to be the case in older communities. Frequent visits from the 'extended family', that is grandchildren, nieces and nephews, sons-in-law and daughters-in-law, help to keep the aged interested in the events of the day.

There is now a great recognition of the ability and willingness of some older people to continue working. Many firms now reserve some jobs especially for older employees whom they find reliable and conscientious and often very methodical workers. Some employers arrange for shorter working hours and sheltered working conditions. It is difficult for some older people to accept positions of less responsibility, with lower status and pay, than those to which they have been accustomed. Many, however, make an excellent adjustment and are glad to postpone complete retirement.

Theory of Disengagement

The older person's method of adjustment is sometimes referred to as 'disengagement'. The ageing person disengages himself by reducing the number of interactions he has with others and by reducing the number of roles he plays in society. He also does so by reducing his life space. Long journeys, which he might have enjoyed earlier in life, are no longer contemplated. He no longer feels he can visit relatives or friends who live a long way away and he shops only in his immediate neighbourhood.

Old people also disengage themselves emotionally. They no longer feel as intensely about events as they did during maturity and this may allow them to develop an attitude of detached tolerance where they might formerly have become angry or hurt. This emotional disengagement may earn the old person a reputation of broadmindedness which often surprises those who were acquainted with him during an

earlier period of strong emotional expression. Emotional disengagement allows the elderly to accept the death of contemporaries with equanimity.

Old age is the time when there is an increasing tendency to
look backwards and to be aware that the future is short.
Planning ahead is normally the most exciting and most
stimulating part of life. Planning a holiday, work, a visit to
friends are important considerations to most people. When
we are very young plans for the future are vague and unrealistic because the future appears infinitely long. Later in
adulthood, planning is realistic and down to earth. There
are short-term and long-term plans, plans concerning the
individual's own future, plans for others or for the development of the daily sphere of action. Only on rare occasions in
adult life may one suddenly realise that these plans may not
come to fruition. When a young friend dies at the height of his
powers or when a dangerous venture is about to be undertaken, for example an operation or a flight, the healthy adult
suddenly thinks of death. But this is momentary and does not
interfere with any long-term plans.

Old people are aware that they may die before plans can be
fulfilled. Consequently less thought is given to the future and
there is a great tendency to live in the present and in the past.
Life becomes somewhat disorganised if there is too much
concentration on the present. Houses are not redecorated or
gardens replanted, new clothes are not bought or holidays
arranged by those who believe they may not live to enjoy the
results. The house, garden and clothes become shabby and the
old person becomes more and more detached and isolated
from others and finally loses any sense of purpose or self-
respect. It is the duty of the younger people to include the
older generation in their plans. Talking of the future, though
not of the very distant future, is a great help. It may be useful to
help the old person to realise how much there is still to be done,

how much to be enjoyed and that it should all be done soon.

If the younger people show by their attitude that they are confident of the older person's future, active old age becomes possible. Inevitably, however, the time must come when the older person thinks of death and must accept the fact that the future is limited—at any rate on this earth. To many people the thought of unlimited life after death and their general religious beliefs are of an importance which cannot be overstressed.

The thought of dying is often more uncomfortable to the young than the old; often, therefore, the old person's attempt to discuss death is pushed aside, even ridiculed. It is not helpful to deny the possibility of death or to deprive the old person of the opportunity of talking of it. Old people die more contentedly if all is in order: if a will has been made, if they can be certain that their property will be well disposed of, that their family is provided for, that all arrangements are made for the burial. To discuss these matters freely and openly need not imply that death is imminent or that the younger one wishes the old person dead. On the contrary, guilt feelings about these wishes often prevent younger people from discussing death.

By the time old age has arrived the prospect of completing life is not usually terrifying. It is made easier if the younger people succeed in conveying to the old their admiration of their past achievement and a determination to carry on where they have left off.

SUGGESTIONS FOR FURTHER READING

BROMLEY, D. B. *The Psychology of Human Ageing*. Harmondsworth: Penguin Books, 1966.

CHOWN, S. M. *Human Ageing*. Harmondsworth: Penguin, 1972.

CUMMING, E. and HENRY, W. E. *Growing Old*. New York: Basic Books, 1961.

LOWE, G. R. *The Growth of Personality from Infancy to Old Age*. Harmondsworth: Penguin, 1972.

8. ATTITUDES TO SICKNESS

To most people illness comes as an unwelcome intrusion. It is a nuisance, an obstacle in the pursuit of some aim in life.

Some people, however, regard illness as a challenge. Their efforts to overcome illness and weakness may lead to greater achievements than would otherwise have been possible. The term 'compensation' is sometimes used to indicate the mechanism of overcoming a weakness. Some patients exercise weak muscles until they become stronger than they would ever have been without the illness. Others, realising that perhaps the leg muscles are weak and will never be able to become very strong, exercise shoulders and arms, learn to move skilfully by using new sets of muscles and to excel in sports and games where the arms can be used, such as archery. Some people use their period of illness for study and reading, develop new interests and gain in education. Suffering helps many people to find a new faith in religion, to discover their purpose in life. Illness can be turned into an asset, helping the development of most desirable characteristics.

Regression

Many people's attitude to illness is much less constructive and many nursing problems arise because sick people often behave not as adults but as if they were much younger. Sickness represents to them a 'stress situation'. Under stress people often revert to earlier patterns of behaviour, they 'regress'. This chapter is concerned mainly with those attitudes to sickness which are determined by childhood memories, by irrational fears and by unexpressed anger. Sickness often causes changes in behaviour which are quite irrational. The patient cannot help himself because he is reacting unconsciously and some of his troubles lie in the past rather than in the current illness.

In previous chapters we have described the stages of development through which children pass, but at no time did we concern ourselves with the way they 'ought' to behave. The psychologist describes, but he does not judge. In this chapter, when we try to understand the behaviour of people who are ill, we again refrain from judging how adults ought to behave.

The Stigma of Illness

In our modern age attitudes to sickness have largely been modified and are to a much less extent than formerly coloured by disgust and rejection. Some illnesses, however, still bear a stigma. People suffering from mental disorders, from epilepsy, from tuberculosis or from venereal diseases are still occasionally treated as outcasts of society. Many people attach value judgments to the concept of health. Physical and mental health are looked upon as good, desirable and praiseworthy. Ill health is often looked upon as a punishment, in many cultures it is regarded as shameful and wicked. Looking upon illness as if it were blameworthy causes sick people to behave with resentment.

It is certainly not at all uncommon for people to adopt this attitude of guilt and shame towards their own sufferings,* so much so that they find it impossible to discuss the illness even with a doctor or nurse. Anyone who thinks badly of himself tends to believe that other people share this attitude. Some people conclude that everybody shuns them and looks at them with disgust, suspicion or disapproval. In the extreme form this attitude is found among those mentally ill people who believe that they 'smell', that they are, covered with 'germs',

* It is interesting to remember that our word *pain* probably comes from the Greek ποινή which means penalty.

or that they emit 'harmful rays'. These patients, consequently, cut themselves off from society believing themselves to be unwanted and a danger to others. In less extreme forms this attitude is very frequently found among all types and classes of men and women. The general practitioner is aware of the fact that some patients are reluctant to come to him and often delay seeking advice until the condition has deteriorated too far. They attempt to deny their illness because they feel it is unacceptable.

Health visitors meet people who simply will not accept care or advice because they cannot admit to being ill. It is strange that certain illnesses are much more frequently hidden or hushed up than others because the feeling of guilt is more marked. Sometimes the guilt feeling appears almost rational and associated with the belief that the illness could have been prevented. Tuberculosis, for example, is often believed to be the result of unhealthy living, irregular hours, scanty food, all of which might have been prevented with proper care. Scabies or infestation is often considered to be the result of dirt and, although infestation can occur in spite of all hygienic precautions, patients feel guilty.

The attitude to venereal disease shows how much our moral judgment is tied up with attitude to illness. Here it is partially rational; on the other hand, when women refuse to consult a doctor about a lump in the breast, a vaginal discharge, or pruritus vulvae, the connection between sex and illness becomes less rational and the feeling of guilt more disturbing. The fear and shame about mental disorder show irrational attitudes in their most highly developed form. Because early diagnosis and treatment are important the patient's feeling of guilt and shame must be taken into account by those who meet people in the early stages of their illness. Nurses working in the community have a great chance to eradicate these harmful attitudes among the general public, among the prospective patients whom they meet in clinics and homes and particularly among their own colleagues.

Guilt Feelings about Illness

Often people believe that illness is a punishment for some misdeed. Some patients who feel guilty look upon the illness as a punishment they deserve; others feel that they are unjustly treated or wonder what they have done to deserve suffering.

The idea of illness being a form of punishment is very frequently expressed in words, either by patients themselves or by anxious relatives who keep assuring themselves and the nurses of the injustice which is being visited upon the patient. The idea that illness is punishment for bad behaviour is found quite naturally in the small child. A mother may, for instance, repeatedly tell the child not to get his feet wet. On one occasion she says, 'If you step into the puddle I'll smack you'; on another occasion, 'If you step into the puddle you'll catch a cold'. What more natural than that catching cold and being smacked are regarded as alternative forms of punishment? In fact, some illnesses are the natural consequences of foolish actions and the parental threat may be good health education. Some deficiency diseases, for example, may follow inadequate food intake, road accidents may follow careless play in the street and later in life follow careless driving.

Unfortunately, there is a tendency to regard any illness as a punishment even when it is unavoidable and in no way attributable to individual negligence or wickedness. One way of helping the patient to overcome these feelings is to encourage free conversation about the subject, dealing with it in a factual way. The nurse's accepting, unemotional attitude to the discussion of illness and her acceptance and understanding of the patient's feelings will do much to reassure him.

When patients or relatives adopt the attitude that the illness must be regarded as punishment and seek to find the guilt for which the punishment has fallen upon them, they adopt an outlook which is not conducive to recovery. Some patients who look at illness as a form of punishment react to it by becoming resentful, angry, rebellious; others by becoming submissive, apologetic or passive.

If the patient regards his illness as punishment he may easily begin to look for someone responsible for his suffering. Some patients turn to God and derive comfort from experiencing God's special interest. Some patients associate the people concerned with the illness with the idea of punishment. They see the ward sister or matron, the nurse carrying out treatment or the doctor as people to be feared and respected. Often the attitude of submission to hospital staff is quite unrealistic. Some of the rules which patients talk about do not really exist: for instance, fear of the ward sister, which is so often expressed by patients and visitors, may have nothing to do with the sister's real personality. Some treatments are more commonly associated with the idea of punishment than others. Surgery, injections, tube feeding, enemata and tests involving electricity, such as electrocardiograms, often give rise to phantasies of punishment with all the appropriate reactions of fear and submission or resentment. Any treatment which renders the patient helpless, for example, by immobilisation of limbs or by causing unconsciousness, may increase his feelings of being punished. Patients do not often express these feelings to the nurse, but their attitude to illness or treatment gives an indication of them. In retrospect patients are sometimes more able to express how they felt and dreams and nightmares sometimes show the connection between the treatment and the phantasy of being punished.

Whenever people are ill and receiving treatment and nursing care they must, to some extent, give up independence and submit to the authority of doctors and nurses. In many respects their position resembles that of a child who is looked after by his mother. Once again, just as in childhood, the patient is relieved of responsibility but at the same time deprived of freedom of action. Someone cares for him just as his mother did once. Once again he experiences tenderness and love but at the same time the frustration of having to do as he is told and of being childishly dependent. The patient sometimes reacts to this situation by using the type of behaviour which he found useful in childhood. Nurses may become targets for hostility and criticism or may receive the patient's complete trust, so much so that at times it may be embarrassing to an inexperienced nurse.

The Need for Attention

Attitude towards illness and towards the person who helps the patient to get well is often learnt in childhood. When the nurse meets the patient in hospital she often sees a repetition of this early pattern.

Some children find that in illness they gain sympathy and attention which is denied them when they are well. In adulthood there is still the feeling that one is entitled to special consideration during illness. Children discover quite early what kind of behaviour is most effective. Crying, moaning, complaining may help some children. Others gain the admiration of their parents by their patience and fortitude. Adult patients use well-tried behaviour patterns quite unconsciously. Some moan, cry, complain and display their suffering; others appear to be able to tolerate a great deal of discomfort without complaint. Sometimes they succeed in gaining special consideration just as they did in childhood. Often the behaviour appears misplaced and fails to fulfil its purpose. Crying and complaining may result only in irritating the nurse or in discouraging visitors, remaining too silent may result in being ignored by a busy staff, but childhood patterns of behaviour may persist even when they turn out to be of no practical use.

All sick people need attention, but their method of seeking it may not be appropriate. Some nurses find it irritating when patients make their need for attention known too forcefully. Nurses often describe patients as 'attention seeking' and they may appear to believe that there is something undesirable about attention-seeking behaviour.

It is helpful to assume that any patient who seeks attention really needs it. Often, when it is freely given and when it is given before the patient has had to ask for it, the 'attention-seeking' behaviour decreases dramatically. If nurses ignore patients who are 'attention seeking' insecurity is increased and needs for attention become even greater. If the need for attention is understood childish attitudes can more easily give way to more adult forms of adaptation.

SUGGESTIONS FOR FURTHER READING

BURTON, G. *Nurse and Patient*. London: Tavistock, 1965.

GOFFMAN, E. *Stigma*. Harmondsworth: Penguin, 1968.

MCGHEE, Mrs A. *The Patient's Attitude to Nursing Care*. Edinburgh: Livingstone, 1961.

ROSE, A. M. *Human Behaviour and Social Processes*. London: Routledge and Kegan Paul, 1962.

SELYE, H. *The Stress of Life*. London: Longmans, 1957.

STOCKWELL, F. *The Unpopular Patient*. London: Royal College of Nursing, 1972.

9. ADMISSION TO HOSPITAL

Admission to hospital causes anxiety and fear in most people. All nurses are aware of the need to do everything in their power to help a new patient to settle down quickly and to carry out admission procedure as encouragingly and reassuringly as possible. To succeed in this it is necessary to try to understand the patient's anxiety and to detect the signs of it. Only a few patients express their worries openly. Many are unable to do so because they are not clearly aware of their worries themselves.

Patients' Needs

People feel comfortable and relaxed when all their physiological and psychological needs have been satisfied. The physiological needs of food, water, warmth are usually satisfied in health. In sickness difficulty in breathing or thirst are always accompanied by anxiety which is easily recognisable.

The psychological needs of the patient are less easily identified. People need to feel secure in their environment. They must understand it and must understand the part they themselves play in it. They need to love and be loved, to be respected and to respect themselves. They need to feel that they are able to master the situation in which they find themselves. None of these needs can be fully satisfied on admission to hospital.

The Need for Security

Security means the ability to predict what is going to happen and how to make things happen. Hospital routine gives security to nurses and later in the patient's stay it gives great security to him also. On arrival, however, he knows nothing at all of the events which are to follow. People around him move, appear busy, do things to him, but he feels completely bewildered and left out of it. His greatest anxiety occurs in relation to his own behaviour. He does not know what is expected of him, what will happen if he does not behave as he is supposed to. He does not know in which way he can influence events, what is the procedure for obtaining attention, whether it is permissible to get out of bed or how to address the nurses who attend to him. His insecurity is all the greater because he finds it difficult to distinguish one nurse from another. It is always difficult to remember people and their names when many new people are met simultaneously and it is all the more confusing when all wear the same uniform.

Anxiety due to lack of security can be alleviated by keeping the patient fully informed of what is going on. Nurses often tell the patient what *they* are going to do but the patient is concerned only with himself. It is more helpful to tell the patient what *he* is going to do and what precisely is going to happen to him, how he is going to experience the events around him.

It is a mistake to tell the patient too much at a time and to give too many explanations on admission. Because of his anxiety he may be unable to pay attention or to remember much of what he is told. If he knows what is going to happen, but not when, he becomes increasingly anxious while he waits and wonders. Explanations are best given in the form of a running commentary as events in the ward take place.

Some information about the geography of the ward, times for meals, the routine of the day, can be given early even if it is not remembered at once. The fact that the nurse is willing to give information is in itself reassuring. Some hospitals give this information in the form of a pamphlet. This has been shown to make the patient feel happy in the knowledge that the hospital cares about him and it makes him feel important. It may, however, also be an indication that the nurses do not wish to be bothered and represent a way of giving information without taking into account what the patient really wants to know or whether he has clearly understood. Personal communication has great advantages.

Specific information should be given only when the patient asks for it. Before this he must be helped to feel that the nurses are willing to be asked, are reliable and interested and have sufficient time to pay attention to his needs. There is usually a phase of testing in which the patient asks several nurses the same question, or asks the same nurse many times over. He may ask about trivialities without listening to the answer. These actions are not deliberate attempts to be difficult. They are symptoms of anxiety; and they serve the purpose of finding the particular nurse who, by her manner, gives him the impression of being the right person with whom to discuss really important matters.

Anxiety may manifest itself in some of the bodily symptoms presented by the patient. Rapid pulse, flushing or pallor of the face, tremor, sweating, widely dilated pupils, dry mouth, nausea, diarrhoea, raised blood pressure, headaches are all symptoms which occur in anxiety. These may mislead the doctor in making his diagnosis and it is therefore very important to help the patient to lose anxiety symptoms as soon as possible. If the patient feels anxious and apprehensive he is unable to concentrate, fails to appreciate the books and magazines offered to him, starts many activities without completing them, asks for many things he does not really want.

He can be helped if there is one special person whom he can recognise, who devotes her time to him and comes to him. Introduction to *one* person is important. This can be the patient in the next bed or one particular nurse or a domestic assistant, one person who represents stability in the chaotic new world into which he has entered. Nurses often wear name badges and this is useful and helps the patient to remember her name. It is no substitute, however, for personal introductions. The nurse should say her name clearly and distinctly and may have to repeat it several times before the patient can use it with confidence. When the patient arrives in hospital he is already at a disadvantage as far as remembering names is concerned. The nurse may already know the name of the patient she is expecting, she can address the patient by name and she expects the patient to spell his name out clearly enough to enter it in the records. The patient does not know the nurses' names and it is important that learning them should be made easy for him.

Although the patient also needs to know which nurse is in charge of the ward, which one is a staff nurse and which ones are student nurses, it is insufficient if the nurse introduces herself by saying: 'I am a student nurse in this ward.' It is much easier for the patient if she says: 'My name is Mary X...; I am a student nurse.' And this introduction should precede the use of the patient's name.

Nurses often believe that the patient's anxiety is primarily related to his disease or his worry about the home situation. This may not be so on admission. There may be a very real cause for alarm yet the patient cannot give his thoughts to the big problem confronting him while he is learning to understand the little problems around him. His most urgent task is getting to know his new environment. Reassurance must, therefore, be concerned with the patient's immediate need to orientate himself adequately in his new surroundings. To refer to the family, the work, the financial matters before the patient has done so is far from reassuring. In fact it may well add to his anxiety and make him feel guilty about his selfishness in thinking of himself.

Trust in the Staff

While the understanding of events and routine helps in creating security, confidence in people is the most important aspect of feeling safe. When the patient is newly admitted his general state of bewilderment is such that he is desperately in need of people and therefore in the best possible position to develop confidence in staff.

The greater people's needs are the more inclined they are to accept help without questioning the competence of those who offer it. A healthy person may critically discuss the relative excellence of several doctors or nurses, but an ill one accepts without question the ministrations of whoever is at hand to give help and assumes that that person is capable of giving care. This phase of uncritical acceptance is an important and valuable factor in initiating treatment. The nurse's manner, her ability to remain calm in the face of the patient's anxiety, her confidence in herself and in her colleagues helps the patient to believe that his trust in the hospital is well founded.

Later during the patient's stay in hospital, as he becomes more secure and settled, he is better able to compare staff, to use rational criteria for assessing the nurses and to become more critical of the people around him. Confidence in nurses, then, must be created by the quality of service which is given to him and which he observes being given to others. Nothing undermines confidence in staff more rapidly than to notice lack of attention to detail in the care of other people.

During the phase in which a patient accepts unquestioningly that doctors, nurses and treatments are good he is said to be highly suggestible. His own judgments are in abeyance, other people's are accepted. It is very important indeed for the nurse to be fully aware of the impact of all she says to a patient at a time like this and to learn how to use voice, gestures and words in such a way that they suggest comfort, hope, progress and optimism. Patients usually seem to prefer the nurse who was present at the time of admission. This may be because she is the only one clearly recognisable in the general chaos which surrounds the patient and the one accepted most uncritically. All the more important that during the admission formalities the nurse should be fully aware of the responsibility her position carries.

Sudden admission to hospital, for example after an accident, may result in anxieties even more inappropriate than those normally observed on admission. People tend to worry about tasks which are not completed and to think about them until they are finished. Everybody has the urge to finish what he is doing and enjoys the satisfaction of seeing the job done. It is difficult, for example, to put a book away in the middle of a chapter or to stop knitting in the middle of a row. Nurses like to stay on until all the beds are made or all temperatures are taken. Lecturers like to feel they have covered all the ground. If anyone is suddenly stopped in the middle of a task he experiences an urge to return to it. Patients suddenly admitted to hospital worry about the things they were about to do. A letter which was meant to be posted, a telephone call, an appointment, a planned visit to a theatre, the fact that his desk has not been tidied up—all these can be of utmost importance to a patient when he is suddenly taken off to hospital, so important in fact that he may refuse to remain in hospital if it is in his power to refuse.

Some patients after road accidents are particularly worried about papers or documents they may have in their possession and cannot accept help for themselves until they know that their papers are taken care of. Pet animals left at home, children who may be expecting mother back, a saucepan left boiling on the stove may cause intense anxiety to the patient who is suddenly taken to hospital.

Patients may have a great need to talk about the accident in which they were involved. Although it may appear upsetting at the time it is better to talk it over and to relive the emotional impact of the accident by talking about it than to try to forget. Nightmares may be recurrent and delayed emotional reaction may be severe if the patient cannot gain a listener's ear soon after the accident.

It may be obvious to the nurse that the patient has more important troubles that he could or should worry about, but what appears trivial to others may seem of the utmost urgency to the patient. It is useless to say, 'Don't worry about that now.' No one can stop worrying when commanded to do so, nor can worries be postponed. Problems must be resolved and the nurse is the person to resolve these urgent difficulties for the patient.

Self-esteem

When the patient feels secure in the hospital he becomes more aware of his other psychological needs. The need to be appreciated, loved and to think well of himself, the need to be of use to others becomes very important. It is difficult for the patient to think well of himself when in a helpless state. The attitudes adopted by the staff and relatives may help, particularly if the patient expresses his fear of being a burden and useless, by apologising for the trouble he is giving or worrying about the fact that he needs attention. The more helpless the illness renders the patient the more his self-esteem needs to be boosted. Incontinence is a symptom which is particularly distressing and so is the need for bedpans, the need to be fed or washed or lifted. The more the nurse has to do for the patient the more she must remember to assure him of her respect so that he can respect himself.

Adolescent patients may find the experience of hospitalisation particularly damaging to their self-esteem. Having only recently established his independent status the young person may find it humiliating to have bodily needs attended to by nurses not much older than himself. It is always humiliating to have one's weaknesses exposed. In illness all weaknesses become known to doctors and nurses; not only those which are symptomatic of the illness which has caused admission to hospital, but also all those weaknesses one has learnt to hide effectively from others, e.g. deformities or skin blemishes. In the process of taking the patient's medical history the doctor learns many intimate details of the patient's life which the patient perhaps discloses only reluctantly. Nurses who take the patient's particulars on admission find out about many personal circumstances which he may perhaps have preferred to keep to himself. To enable a patient to retain his self-esteem, when so many circumstances combine to rob him of it, is one of the most important functions of a nurse. It helps to allow the patient to tell his story in his own way without too many interruptions. The order in which the patient offers the information indicates which points seem important to him. The list of questions on the patient's record form should be regarded as a check list to ensure that all necessary details have been recorded, but to insist that the patient give name, address and next of kin when he is trying to explain a matter of greater concern to him gives the impression of belittling his anxiety and reduces his self-esteem.

When the patient begins to express concern about the welfare of his family he may wish to return to his position of responsibility as soon as possible. While a realistic appreciation of the family's welfare is a good sign the patient's anxiety is sometimes not so much for his family as an expression of his fear that he might not be as necessary to them as he had thought. Every family must adjust itself to the sickness of one of its members. Work and responsibilities have to be re-allocated so that the least suffering is caused to all concerned. The patient's place in the family circle is not left wide open, the gap is filled by one or more members of the family who assume the responsibilities of the absent member.

The patient may begin to realise that the family can do without him. He may be glad and yet upset by his loss of status. He may worry about them to convince himself that he is really needed and may not be at all reassured by being told that all is well. The same feelings occur in relation to work; an unconscious fear that he may not be indispensable after all and an increased preoccupation with all the work he ought to be doing.

It is difficult for the nurse to help the patient to feel important in relation to his family. Visitors can be helped to see the need to increase the patient's feeling of participation in outside affairs. The patient's self-esteem can be raised within the hospital by asking for his help with other patients, asking his advice, making him feel he belongs. Conversation about home and work is important as soon as the patient is able to think of it. The nurse should remember that the patient derives no help from being told not to concern himself with the problems of others. His rehabilitation becomes increasingly difficult the more he has detached himself from his former ties.

The Need to be Independent

During the patient's recovery his independence and his need for mastery become more pronounced. While at first he may be content to let events run their course and merely try to understand them his return to health makes him feel that he needs to be able to influence and change events if he wishes. He begins to ask questions about his treatment, expresses doubts, asks for explanations. He begins to remind nurses that his medicine is due or to tell them how he wishes treatment carried out. He may begin to ignore rules, to refuse to eat the prescribed diet or to smoke though it is not permitted. This growing independence is a most encouraging sign of improvement. Just as children learn gradually to become independent so the patient too takes one step at a time, waiting to see what the results of his initiative may be. Part of this process results in a better knowledge of other people's individual reactions. Patients, like children, learn when it is safe to break rules and when it is not, which members of the staff become hurt or bad-tempered when contradicted or reminded of something, which appear to welcome help and encourage independence. Just like children patients may try to see how far they can go without disrupting the environment before they can settle and assume responsibility for their own action, bearing in mind the needs of others.

The more secure the staff feel in their ability to maintain the right atmosphere and to satisfy the individual needs of each patient the more they encourage a return to independence as soon as the patient is ready.

SUGGESTIONS FOR FURTHER READING

FRANKLIN, B. L. *Patient Anxiety on Admission to Hospital.* London: Royal College of Nursing, 1974.

MUNDAY, A. *Physiological Measures of Anxiety in Hospital Patients.* London: Royal College of Nursing, 1973.

10. THE PATIENT'S FAMILY

Sickness always has far-reaching effects on the patient's family. Even a mild, short illness in the patient's own home causes marked emotional reactions.

In the early stages of the illness the patient may be reluctant to give in and, though clearly unwell, he tries to continue his activities. His family feels concern, sympathy and solicitude and tries to persuade him to allow himself to be looked after. Gradually, however, his relatives may experience irritation at the patient's obstinacy and withdraw sympathy just at the moment when the patient, unconsciously perhaps, begins to enjoy the concern people show for him. When eventually the patient is forced to give up both he and his family may feel guilty about their previous attitudes. The family may feel that they have not taken the symptoms sufficiently seriously and the patient may have begun to feel doubtful about the support his family is able to give.

If the patient is to be nursed at home considerable stress may arise. There is much extra work, which is worrying to the patient who has caused it and is often resented by the family. In prolonged illness this is often realised. In the early period of sickness the members of the family are, however, unable to admit their resentment and their guilt feeling about it may make them behave as if they were martyrs, doing much more work than necessary and depriving themselves of all opportunity to rest or take time off away from the patient.

Patients who are not ill enough to be admitted to hospital are often able to retain more independence than hospitalised patients. This may make nursing difficult as the patient may refuse to obey doctor's orders, may get up though not permitted to do so, refuse treatment or drugs and may feel that he should retain some say in the management of the home. The relationship between the patient and the relative who nurses him is to some extent maintained at the normal adult level, but the patient also reacts to being nursed as he would if he were in hospital by becoming helpless and dependent. Relatives are less able than nurses to enforce a therapeutic régime, partly because of the dual role, partly because they tend to become too worried about the patient's illness.

Nurses are often better able to assist than relatives because they are not too emotionally involved. Though she cares very much for the patient's welfare the nurse's private life and emotional balance are not affected by his progress, be it favourable or not. Relatives cannot avoid being involved. To them the patient's recovery or deterioration is a matter of personal concern. Their joy or anxiety about his condition is bound to affect his progress.

One of the problems of nursing a member of the family is the reluctance of the patient to allow relatives to carry out any intimate nursing care or to let them see him in any condition in which he would not normally allow himself to be seen. Patients and relatives may feel embarrassed about the use of bedpans, disposal of vomit, changing bedclothes or personal hygiene. This may result in inadequate care, either because the patient may be reluctant to ask for help or because the relative cannot overcome his repugnance at nursing the patient.

Prolonged illness in the home very often results in increasing isolation of the family as a whole. Visiting by friends tends to be frequent at first, but after some time people find the company of invalids distressing and they eventually withdraw. The family who is busy nursing an invalid becomes uninteresting to others and is increasingly ostracised. Although help or relief may be urgently needed it may be difficult to take the initiative of making the need known and the result may be bitterness and hostility. There is also often the additional expense of entertaining visitors, which may result in considerable financial sacrifice.

When the patient is admitted to hospital the family's difficulties may be even more considerable. It may result in increased work in the home, depending on the patient's position in the family. In any case complete reorganisation of routine is necessary. If the breadwinner is in hospital financial worries may be added to those resulting from sickness. If the mother is away children may have to be cared for by neighbours or distant relatives. Details of family life which have been kept strictly private become known to relative strangers. Members of the family become aware of and fear criticism, even if it is not voiced, of the way in which the home is run, the children brought up and personal affairs managed. If it is necessary to obtain financial assistance details about family life must be disclosed which hitherto may not even have been known to all members of the family.

Visiting in hospital is a major problem for patients and relatives. Patients look forward to visiting time and yet often find it disappointing when it happens. There may be so many visitors that the patient is unable to establish contact with any of them. He may find visiting too tiring and still feel he should make the effort to take an interest. If visitors are late or if the patient is without visitors he becomes angry and distressed and then finds his visitors even less satisfying when they do arrive. Relatives often find visiting a great strain. If visiting hours are infrequent they may have the greatest difficulty in being free just at the time when visiting is allowed and may find it difficult to arrange for all those who would like to visit to be able to take a turn. If visiting is short and frequent they may feel obliged to come each time, which may be most upsetting to family routine. If the journey is long it is very difficult to time the departure from home in such a way as to arrive on time. Whichever way visiting is arranged relatives feel worried by the time they arrive in hospital, they worry about the visit itself, worry about the patient's condition. Uncertainty about the way in which they can obtain information and the feeling that information may be incomplete may add to their troubles. The visiting period passes quickly and relatives may share with the patient a feeling of disappointment and dissatisfaction about their contact. It is difficult to be affectionate in an open ward. There is usually a time-lag before emotional rapprochement can be made and the number of interruptions makes it more difficult.

Separation of children from their parents can cause great anxiety to all concerned. The importance of visiting children frequently when they are ill is discussed in another chapter. When mother is ill it may be a great comfort if children are occasionally allowed to see her. The mother often worries quite unnecessarily about the welfare of her children at home and is reassured when she sees them. Children share in all the anxiety which is associated with the illness of the mother. They may find it difficult to imagine what hospital is like; they may not be able to believe that mother is really ill unless they can see her in bed in hospital; they may have phantasies about her having died and fail to be reassured by those who have been to visit her. Very young children, especially, experience a great sense of loss and emptiness when mother is not with them and explanations cannot satisfy them. Visits should be arranged if it is at all possible. However emotionally difficult a reunion followed by renewed separation may be to adults and to the children, the long-term effects are beneficial to all. It is usually not as difficult to prevent children's noise as is often feared and the children are so intent on the visit to their mother that they can easily be distracted from any unpleasant sights which might be thought to upset them.

Many visitors find conversation with the patient very difficult. They ask the patient questions about the way he feels and what is happening to him. If the patient is fairly ill he cannot answer adequately. If he is well enough to talk he does not have much news to tell and in any case should not be expected to keep on talking about his symptoms and treatment or the condition of his neighbours. The patient may become silent and the visitors in their embarrassment turn to each other for conversation. It may be necessary to help visitors to realise that they have much more news to give the patient than the patient has for them. Their reluctance to talk of home or the outside world may be caused by fear of worrying the patient or of making him feel envious of the interesting time they are having. The patient should, however, be kept in touch with what is going on. He has much greater incentive to get well if he knows that he is missed. His return home is made much easier if he is kept fully informed of events. His interest should at times be focused more on other people than on himself. It is all too easy for a patient in hospital to lose interest in the fate of others and to have as his sole topics of conversation himself, the nurses and hospital routine. All the small happenings of the hospital ward become magnified in importance and significance. His preoccupation with the little world of the hospital contributes to his relatives' discomfort when they visit unless they can be induced to break into it by talking about themselves. Relatives may feel reluctant to burden the patient with their own problems, perhaps not realising that it may be more worrying to the patient to feel completely useless than to know that his absence is felt and that he is being consulted.

When relatives experience emotional difficulties about visiting they either find excuses for coming less often or they may attempt to deal with their feelings by becoming critical of the hospital, the treatment and the staff. When this happens they need an opportunity of discussing all their worries about the patient's illness at length with the doctor, the ward sister or the social worker. Nurses may find it difficult to see how they can influence relationships between patients and visitors. They may feel uncomfortable at visiting times and take the opportunity of disappearing from the ward, therefore depriving themselves of a most prolific source of information about the patient and of an opportunity to help him. Information about the patient's condition can, of course, be given only by one person. If all the nurses were permitted to do this conflicting or inaccurate information might be passed on. This should not, however, prevent nurses from talking freely to the patient's visitors. It is helpful to visitors to be recognised, to be greeted in a friendly manner and to exchange with the nurses a few words about the way the patient has been passing his time. For example the nurse might say: 'Your husband enjoyed the jigsaw puzzle you brought him'; or to a mother: 'Johnnie was playing with his toy cars this morning'. This kind of information is appreciated because it indicates the nurse's interest. It is a conversational opening which might help the visitor to speak to the nurse about anything that worries her and it could be an opening remark which could facilitate conversation between the patient and his visitors.

The nurse's presence at visiting time may, moreover, be helpful in discovering when relatives feel uncomfortable or worried. The fact that the nurse knows who has visited the patient may help him to talk about his feelings in relation to his family. It may be possible to mention to the relatives that the patient is interested in their news.

It is usual for visitors to take some present to a patient in hospital. Nearly always they bring food. This is partly tradition, partly it results from the widely held belief that hospital food is bad and partly from the fact that social convention suggests gifts of food to indicate love for the patient. Although hospital food is usually quite good and adequate patients appreciate anything which is brought in by visitors.

The association of food with people one likes is so strong that food tastes quite different when it is offered by someone whom the patient loves. Even though food may not be needed it is unwise to tell visitors not to bring it in as they and the patient feel the need for a tangible exchange of gifts. Nurses should not feel any implied criticism in the fact that relatives enjoy giving pleasure to the patient. If too much of the wrong kind of food accumulates it is more helpful to make positive suggestions as to what might be brought instead than to tell the patient's relatives not to bring anything. A suggestion to bring the patient something to do may occasionally be helpful. Puzzles, amusing pictures, books, paints, magazines, photographs, needlework may help the patient to regain interest. Many relatives fail to appreciate this when they visit adult patients.

When the patient is critically ill and visiting is unrestricted the conflict in the relatives is often at its maximum. There is a feeling that the patient ought not to be left, combined with a sense of helplessness and uselessness that makes visiting extremely painful. All nurses are aware of the intense emotion which arises while visitors are at or near the bedside of a patient on sick notice. The greatest comfort for the visitor is activity. Whenever relatives can assist in doing something for the patient or be of some use in the ward they feel very much better. There is a widespread belief that the ward must always be in perfect order before visiting time and that visitors should leave whenever any attention is given to the patient, but there is no proof that this is at all helpful to the visitor. It is much easier for the visitor to appreciate how well a patient is being nursed when he is allowed to witness some of the procedures or even to give a helping hand.

It is always difficult to decide how much to tell when a patient is seriously ill. Often the doctor tells the relative but not the patient thus putting a tremendous burden on the relative who tries his utmost to remain cheerful and optimistic when talking to the patient. Often the patient knows, even if he has not been told, how serious his illness is but he tries to hide it from the relatives. Both may long to speak of their anxiety but be afraid to do so. Responsibility for giving information rests with the doctor, but the nurse is the person who becomes aware of the tension which results from attempts to hide feelings and she is also the one who can assist patients and relatives to find someone in whom each can confide.

Discharge from hospital requires a reorganisation in the home and reorientation of the patient's interest. The whole family needs time to prepare and an opportunity to sort out their feelings about each other and about their position in the community as a whole. Sudden discharge may be as upsetting as sudden admission to hospital. Whenever possible ample time should be given to the family and every help to the patient to prepare himself for separation from the hospital and for resumption of his role in the family.

11. CHRONIC SICKNESS AND INVALIDISM

When an illness is acute and of short duration the sudden changes in the patient's needs and the rapid reorganisation of family relationships cause difficulties in the care of the patient. Chronic, long-standing illness and permanent disablement create problems of a different nature.

In the course of growing up people develop ideas about themselves which determine how they behave in different situations. They get to know their capabilities and in their daily lives undertake only those activities of which they know themselves to be capable. Interests develop according to individual ability to understand the subject and take an active part. People, for example, compete in sports only when they can approximately equal the performance of others; they study only those subjects which are within their competence and present themselves for examinations only if there is at least a chance of passing. Choice of friends is often determined by mutual interests. Friends are made at work or amongst those who play the same games, share a particular interest, or are equally energetic in climbing mountains.

People's estimate of their own ability usually becomes surprisingly accurate, although some may have been so profoundly discouraged during childhood that they consistently underestimate their ability and lack confidence. Some people who grow up with a handicap devote most of their energy to overcoming it and excel in the use of precisely those skills which they have found hardest to acquire. Others cope with their disability by ignoring it and concentrating on excelling in some other sphere of activity. These methods of compensating for some real or imagined inferiority are part of the driving force in people's way of life. Gradual changes in ability as it increases during growth and declines in old age are incorporated into people's ideas of themselves.

Accepting Disablement

Illness is regarded as a temporary interference in the normal process of life and does not, at first, lead to a change in outlook. Prolonged and chronic illness and permanent disablement, however, necessitate a complete reconstruction of the patient's ideas of himself and a complete reorganisation of relationships. The ordinary expectations of the family and of society as a whole must be changed. This process is slow and painful and requires considerable assistance from those who are nursing the patient.

When the patient first realises that he cannot get completely well he may become depressed. He may feel that in such circumstances life is not worth living. He may lose interest in himself, his treatment and the conditions surrounding him. When the patient is in this frame of mind it is very difficult to nurse him, as he himself does nothing to help. He may refuse to take sufficient nourishment, neglects his personal hygiene, loses all interest in any activity. All nurses know that the will to live is essential to recovery and they must help the patient to see that in spite of his handicap he is needed by those who love him and that he can still be useful to the community.

Stigma

Often the patient who realises that he is permanently disabled becomes furiously angry with himself and with everyone whom he feels he can blame for his predicament. He may express his feeling in his criticism of the treatment and care he is receiving in the hospital, possibly even in litigation against the hospital or those he thinks are responsible for his condition, or he may accuse his family or people in general of being hard-hearted, of disliking him because he is a burden to them, of looking down on invalids. At some stage of the illness most disabled people project their anger onto other people. They refuse to meet people, refuse to be seen or to go out. This phase of self-consciousness increases the difficulties because, while originally people may not have harboured any of the feelings ascribed to them, the patient's attitude creates in them embarrassment, discomfort and eventually rejection.

Difficulty in Communication

It is inevitable that a disabled person must lose some of his former friends. For example if he can no longer play golf he loses interest in the conversation of his golfing friends; if he can no longer work he loses interest in discussion about his former job. After an initial attempt to keep in touch he becomes increasingly isolated from all those whose interests he can no longer share.

The greatest isolation occurs in those who lose sight, hearing or speech. We rely, in our social contacts, on communication by speech and we keep informed about our environment mainly by sight and hearing. It is important for the nurse to learn how to communicate with the deaf by gesture, mime, writing and demonstration, how to help the friends and relatives to continue their efforts to communicate in spite of deafness. She must remember the suspiciousness of the deaf that someone might be talking about them. Partially deaf people may be even more handicapped because they may be less conscious of defective hearing and more inclined to blame others for failing to make themselves clear.

People who have become partially sighted or blind need constant interpretation of their environment while they are learning to use their other senses. It is possible for the nurse to pay more attention to noises and movement and to explain their meaning to the blind person before he becomes startled by someone's presence. The total isolation of those who cannot see may lead to a period of confusion, disorientation and a terrifying feeling of being lost which may result in uncontrolled, sometimes aggressive behaviour.

Patients who cannot speak can make their wishes known by signs and non-articulate noises. It is a great effort for them, however, to attract attention and, having done so, to make themselves clear. It is easy to become impatient with the person who is aphasic but very necessary to take all the time needed to understand. Nurses can learn to anticipate the patient's needs and to save him the effort of trying to speak; each patient's individual language of mime can also be learnt. However, in the long run the patient's speech difficulty may lead other people to stop speaking to him and thus deprive him of intellectual stimulation and social contact. To avoid this every effort should be made to teach the patient new methods of communication.

One-sided conversation may be a very useful way of maintaining contact. The deaf can be encouraged to speak while the nurse merely nods; the aphasic patient can be spoken to and only needs to show his assent or disagreement by nodding.

The nursing care and rehabilitation of the disabled must aim at helping the patient to accept his disability as soon as possible, to create a new idea of himself which includes his handicap. It is sometimes difficult to know how soon the patient should be confronted with the fact that prognosis is not too good. Often, in a well-meaning attempt to spare him suffering, it is not mentioned for a long time. By then the patient has already begun to realise that all is not well and, sensing other people's reluctance to face facts, he keeps his worry to himself and begins to see himself as an object of pity and despair. It may be much wiser to encourage talk of the future as early as possible, and to help the patient to get to know himself as a different, but in no way inferior person to the one he used to be.

Rehabilitation

This can best be done by emphasising what the patient can do rather than what is no longer possible for him. If he has lost the power of his legs he can work with his hands, he can paint or learn a new craft. He can use artificial limbs to perform skills he may never have realised he possessed. It may not be very wise to overemphasise progress in the use of the disabled part of the body. Improved use of the muscles is at the same time a reminder of the deficiency of movement. However helpful physiotherapy, for example, may be it is a constant reminder of disablement. The creation of new interests, new skills in no way connected with the disabled part of the body, gives a positive, purposive direction to life.

Many patients are able first to accept the fact that they may be useful to other sufferers of their own kind. Associations for sufferers from poliomyelitis, paraplegia or epilepsy may, for example, offer the opportunity of doing useful work and of developing the ability to meet people again. Help is more easily accepted from those who are fellow-sufferers because there is no need to feel that help is given only out of pity. There are opportunities of working with other disabled people in special workshops and clubs. Competition in sports can be encouraged. Many paraplegic patients, for example, excel in archery. Many disabled people take an interest in collecting funds for research and for treatment of their illness for the benefit of future patients. Gradually, however, the disabled person must be led to feel equal to though different from other people; able to hold his own in a newly formed circle of friends and fellow workers.

The process of becoming used to the idea of a new and different self must be accompanied by parallel changes in the expectations and attitudes of the family. During the patient's illness it is easy to make allowances for his deficiencies and excuse all he says or does by reference to his condition. This cannot be done for ever, and gradually the family realises that changes in the patient may be permanent. They must learn when to stop considering the patient as the focus of all attention and begin to expect from him a certain amount of consideration.

When the family begins to treat him as a responsible person he may respond by accepting responsibility and becoming interested in living once more as full a life as possible. Some families, of course, find it difficult to readjust themselves to the patient's resumption of his position. The patient's illness may have served as a convenient excuse for them to explain their failure to reach acceptable standards of living. For the patient disablement may be a respectable way of explaining his failure to cope with the stresses of life. When illness is used by the family in this way the whole family is in need of help, support and encouragement.

In the rehabilitation of chronically disabled persons the most difficult task for the nurse is to know when not to help. There is always, on her part, a great temptation to assist those who are fumbling to do things for themselves because she can do them better and more quickly and to relieve people of actions which are obviously painful and difficult for them. It is, however, necessary to let disabled people do as much for themselves and for others as they are able if their self-respect is not to be damaged and their progress impeded. At the same time it must be made as easy as possible for them to ask for help and when it is asked for it must be given in a matter-of-fact way. Help given as an equal in a difficult task is acceptable; help given in such a way as to make the patient feel a passive recipient of care is humiliating.

Much of what is involved in the rehabilitation of the disabled is similar to the way in which we help children to grow up. We encourage every sign of independence, helping only where help must be given, but without making the child feel small or insignificant. All the time the child is growing up he develops new and changing relationships with the people around him until eventually he considers that he is an adult in an adult society, different from all others but with a special contribution to make.

Many chronically disabled people can be helped to return to gainful employment. Sometimes it is necessary for them to change their occupation and undergo a course of training. Some patients may be able to return to their former type of occupation provided they find work in suitable premises, for example, where there is a lift or the work is on the ground floor. Adjustment may have to be made in working hours to allow for rest breaks, or in working conditions to enable the man to carry out his work from his wheelchair or with specially designed equipment. Sympathetic employers may considerably assist rehabilitation or it may be necessary to register for employment under the Disablement Resettlement Acts.

Return to work needs long and careful preparation. It may take many months before a patient is willing to see the disablement resettlement officer, or before he can bear to discuss the possible need for retraining. Close contact between the patient's family and the hospital and between employer and hospital may help the patient considerably. Close co-operation, good communications and complete frankness by all concerned is required during rehabilitation with the emphasis on an optimistic but realistic outlook on life.

Recent legislation ensures that public places, such as theatres and libraries, are now accessible to disabled people and that financial assistance is readily available. These facilities are not, however, always made use of because disabled people are often reluctant to accept the label of 'handicapped person' and the associated experience of feeling stigmatised. A determined educational effort is necessary if the disabled are to participate fully in society.

Deterioration and Death

It is not always possible to achieve improvement. Some conditions are progressive, causing increasing dependence, disablement and suffering. Patients and their relatives are often aware of the unfavourable prognosis before anyone has thought fit to discuss it. Considerable unhappiness and anxiety occurs if this has happened. The patient may feel obliged to pretend that he feels optimistic in order not to cause pain to his relatives. Relatives and friends may believe that a pretence of cheerfulness on their part will spare suffering for the patient.

It is usually very much easier for all concerned to bear the sorrow involved, knowing of the poor prognosis, if they can freely talk to each other, comfort and support each other. The patient may wish to make realistic plans. He may want to have some say in any decisions which are made about him. Where he is to spend the rest of his life is of great concern to him. Hospital wards are not the most desirable environment for prolonged disablement. Young people suffering from chronic illness are particularly unhappy in the chronic, often geriatric, wards of long-stay hospitals. A co-operative effort of friends and family can sometimes enable a patient to spend the remainder of his life in his own home if help can be provided.

Financial assistance may be necessary to provide such aids as wheelchairs or lifting hoists. Structural alterations in the home may be necessary if the stairs are an obstacle to movement or if the doors are too narrow to allow the passage of wheelchairs. Gadgets may have to be bought to help the patient to retain some independence. Special clothing, which can be put on and taken off in spite of the patient's difficulties in movement or posture, may be needed.

Laundry facilities and transport may have to be provided. The family may be able to cope if assistance is available from district nurses or home helps or if it is financially possible for someone to give up paid employment to look after the invalid.

All these arrangements can only be set in motion if the patient and his relatives can freely discuss the problem with each other. Most people find it uncomfortable to talk openly of their thoughts about impending death, but the thought must be faced by relatives and by the patient. If the prognosis is that of a long-drawn-out, gradually deteriorating condition the patient may need to prepare himself for suffering, for a life in which, increasingly, he will be a burden to others. He may have thoughts about suicide, or a wish for euthanasia, which he may need to discuss with someone. He may have plans for the completion of some work and need urgent assistance, he may have some wishes which remain unfulfilled and may wish to tell his relatives about this.

He may wish to prepare himself for death, in a practical manner by putting his affairs in order, and spiritually perhaps with the help of his minister of religion. The patient's reference to dying should certainly not be dismissed lightly. Relatives, too, may need to discuss their feelings when they learn of the adverse prognosis for the patient. Guilt feelings almost inevitably occur. Sometimes a relative may feel the patient's illness could have been prevented if only he had paid attention earlier to the complaints. Some relatives reproach themselves for real or imaginary neglect of the patient. Many relatives become irritable with the patient at times and then feel unhappy about their attitude. The emotional and financial strain of chronic illness often results in a secret wish for a speedy death. Such a wish is followed by immediate regret and by attempts to compensate for the guilt feelings which such a wish arouses. Relatives need someone who can help them to see that such thoughts are normal and understandable. When relatives can talk about their feelings they can often continue to shoulder the burden of caring for an invalid or of visiting frequently. When they cannot talk about their feelings their only remedy may be to detach themselves from the patient prematurely. Decreasing frequency in visiting may be an indication that the relatives behave as if the patient had died already. They cannot bear the pain of witnessing deterioration in their loved one. They mourn the loss of the perfect image of the person they loved and, by the time the patient dies, their grief may already be spent.

Patients and their relatives need assurance that death, when it eventually arrives, will be made as painless as possible. Discussion with the doctor about the problems of dying is often a comfort to all.

Not all patients are upset by witnessing the death of other patients. On the contrary, to observe the peaceful death of another, to witness the support the staff are able to give, to observe the dignified behaviour of the staff in the presence of death, and to know from their behaviour that they care, may make the prospect of dying a good deal less terrifying.

When death eventually occurs grief may need an outward display and the nurse's encouragement in this may be valued. Immediately following a patient's death the relatives may need practical help with initiating funeral arrangements. How people observe the period of mourning is determined by cultural influences. Later on it seems important to many people to have done everything in the correct way. At the time of death it can be the nurse who helps the relatives to sort things out and to begin an adjustment to an altered future.

SUGGESTIONS FOR FURTHER READING

Disabilities and How to Live with Them. London: Lancet Publications, 1952.

GOFFMAN, E. *Stigma*. Harmondsworth: Penguin, 1968.

HINTON, J. *Dying*. Harmondsworth: Penguin, 1967.

QUINT, J. C. *The Nurse and the Dying Patient*. New York: Macmillan, 1967.

RITCHIE, D. *Stroke*. 2nd ed. London, 1966.

WALSH, J. J. *Understanding Paraplegia*. London: Tavistock, 1964.

WINT, GUY. *The Third Killer*. London: Chatto and Windus, 1965.

12. PSYCHOLOGICAL DISORDERS

So far we have concerned ourselves with the effect of illness and hospitalisation on those whose personality development had progressed normally prior to their illness.

Frequently nurses are called upon to care for people whose illness is partly or wholly due to psychological difficulties. The nursing care of psychiatric patients requires special skills, the discussion of which is beyond the scope of this book. Here, only those psychological difficulties which do not necessitate admission to a psychiatric hospital are considered.

In the course of her work in general hospital wards the nurse may meet three broad groups of psychological disorders: patients who suffer from psychosomatic disorders; patients whose symptoms are neurotic; and patients who, in the course of illness, become confused and disorientated. Many nurses find confused, restless patients frightening and need to be reminded that the patient's symptoms are largely the result of his feelings of insecurity. The main contribution the nurse can make to the patient's comfort is to help him to orientate himself. She can try to simplify the environment until the patient can understand it and she can make full use of all those non-verbal methods of communication which the patient may be able to understand.

Psychosomatic Disorders

'Psychosomatic disorders' is the name given to those illnesses in which emotional factors play a major part. Improvement occurs when the patient feels happy and relaxed; exacerbation when the patient is tense and worried.

In all psychosomatic disorders there is physical dysfunction which may require treatment. The treatment remains ineffective, however, if the patient's psychological needs are not met. Asthmatic attacks, for example, occur more frequently in children who are under pressure to work harder at school and often cease when the child changes to another school. During an attack the child needs drugs which are prescribed to relieve spasms. Between attacks care must be taken to avoid exposure to those agents to which he is known to be allergic. Above all the child needs to feel that his potentialities and limitations are recognised and that he is loved in spite of his limitations. If love and recognition are missing treatment fails.

The patient's psychological difficulties usually lie outside the hospital setting. Attitudes towards members of the family may cause an emotional state in which psychosomatic symptoms occur. When the patient is removed to hospital his home problems may recede into the background and symptoms improve only to become worse before, during or after visiting, or as soon as discharge from hospital is envisaged. On the other hand the frustrating feeling of being removed from the scene of difficulties, of being prevented from taking an active part in resolving them, may cause the patient increased anxiety and increased manifestations of symptoms.

Some nurses find it difficult to understand why the patient's symptoms bear no relationship to the care and treatment given in hospital. It is easy to feel angry with the patient, almost as if he were to blame for not responding to treatment. New tensions are then set up which have their origin within the hospital setting and make recovery even more difficult. Generally speaking patients with psychosomatic symptoms respond better to treatment if they can be helped to relax and to free themselves from worry and anxiety. But, as we have already said, worry does not disappear just because the patient is told not to worry. At times it is necessary to resolve difficulties by thinking about them, facing them and actively doing something about them.

The nurse's task lies in reducing causes for anxiety to a minimum within the hospital and in trying to understand the underlying anxiety in the patient's own life. Observation of the patient's reaction to visitors, to the letters he receives, sometimes listening to the patient's stories about his family or work may help her to gain some understanding of his difficulties and will prevent her becoming irritated with the patient and his relatives.

Neurotic Disorders

Some patients are admitted to hospital for investigation of physical complaints which turn out to be neurotic in origin. Some of the symptoms are an exaggeration of anxiety symptoms which can affect any part of the body. The patient may complain of circulatory disturbances such as palpitations, rapid pulse, raised blood pressure, flushing or excessive perspiration. He may have tremors and muscle pain, gastrointestinal disturbances such as nausea or diarrhoea, or urinary dysfunction such as frequency of micturition. The symptoms may become very severe. As the patient goes from doctor to doctor for investigation without any positive diagnosis being reached or any alleviation of symptoms his anxiety becomes focused on the symptoms themselves. He no longer realises that he has these symptoms because he is anxious; instead he feels anxious because he has symptoms. He begins to observe himself and to notice physiological changes. Before long he is labelled as 'hypochondriacal' because he is so preoccupied with his own health. Repeated negative investigations create anxiety in both patient and staff. After initial enthusiasm for making tests the doctor may lose interest when he realises that no organic disorder is present. The doctor's decreasing interest increases the patient's preoccupation with symptoms. A new hospital or a new doctor is sought or a sudden crop of new symptoms starts the cycle of events again.

Sometimes nurses may be heard to say that 'there is nothing wrong with the patient, he is only neurotic'. This kind of thinking is, of course, totally erroneous. The patient has a great deal wrong with him even if his troubles are not organic. His neurotic disorder is more severely disabling than many organic diseases. The patient can be helped if his neurotic disorder is treated positively instead of being dismissed as unimportant. The cause of his anxiety needs to be taken into account. It may be too deep-seated to respond to simple nursing measures. The help of a psychiatrist may be required in order to help the patient to reform his personality pattern, to gain insight into his problems and finally to cope with his feelings of inadequacy.

Meanwhile the patient's hypochondriacal symptoms are the nurse's concern. Emphasis on symptoms is the patient's way of indicating that he needs attention and sympathy. The nurse must acquire the art of convincing the patient that he can gain attention and sympathy more easily by being well than by being ill. She must show her readiness to give care generously without it being asked for, show her enjoyment in the patient's company when he is not complaining, show her solicitude for him though he has no symptoms. When symptoms arise they must be dealt with effectively but unemotionally, quickly before they increase, without making the patient feel guilty about having them and without suggesting more symptoms to the patient.

It would be wrong to say—as may occasionally be heard— that the symptoms should be ignored. Rather, there should be an endeavour to take more interest in the patient than in the symptoms and to allow this interest to reach a climax when the patient is symptom-free. This is difficult enough even when the patient's original symptoms are unrelated to hospital care and more difficult still when the patient reacts to the hospital by producing new symptoms.

Anxiety symptoms manifest themselves in physiological dysfunctions of the autonomic nervous system. Other physical symptoms of a neurotic character are called 'hysterical conversion symptoms'. These symptoms resemble organic disorders of the peripheral or central nervous system. Pain, loss of sensation, blindness, deafness are among the sensory symptoms; paralysis of arm or leg, inability to produce sound, tics, tremors and fits are some of the motor symptoms. A patient who develops hysterical conversion symptoms quite unconsciously solves an emotional conflict by being ill. Having done so he is unaware of his emotional difficulties, denies having any conflict and appears to treat his apparently physical defect with indifference.

A man whose intellectual level may make it difficult for him to hold a skilled, well-paid job, but who feels that it is a disgrace to change to a less demanding occupation, may solve his difficulty by developing a paralysed leg, thus providing himself with a good reason for giving up his work without losing face. A woman may feel furiously angry with her child, longing to hit it, yet feeling guilty about her attitude which she may consider incompatible with maternal love. Paralysis of the arm prevents her hitting the child.

Patients suffering from hysterical conversion symptoms often find their way into general hospital wards for investigation. When organic disorder is excluded they often meet with an attitude of scorn, contempt and irritation. Hysterical symptoms are always purposive. The purpose they serve is never clear to the patient but may be so obvious to others that they find the patient irritating. The patient needs someone to help him solve his conflict so that he no longer needs the symptom. He cannot give up the symptom while his problems remain pressing. The nurse cannot usually help to solve an emotional conflict, but she can try to understand it. She needs to pay attention to the patient himself rather than to his symptoms.

Patients who suffer from neurotic disorders have not learnt to solve their problems in an adult or rational manner. Instead they behave childishly, attempting to gain sympathy by a demonstration of suffering or avoiding action by being sick. Their behaviour in an environment where all the staff are busy and all the patients are preoccupied with themselves can be a source of irritation. Recognition of the patient's need for help, and giving help before the patient resorts to demonstrative symptoms of sickness, can help to establish sufficient confidence to initiate psychiatric treatment if this is necessary.

Care of Suicidal Patients

One of the greatest challenges to the nurse is the care of the patient who has attempted suicide. Because of the physical damage the patient has inflicted upon himself he may be nursed in a general hospital though the desperate nature of his act and the depression which has led him to it makes psychiatric treatment imperative. It is often difficult for one who is happy and contented with life to imagine the intensity of suffering of the depressed patient. Because most nurses—just like most other people—disapprove of suicide and perhaps consider it sinful they may not find it easy to give the patient the sympathy and understanding he needs.

The patient's suicidal attempt indicates the utter loneliness and hopelessness he has experienced. His illness may cause him to suffer from totally unjustified feelings of unworthiness or guilt. His ideas are then said to be 'delusional'. They are none the less real and unbearable to the patient. Alternatively, the feeling of hopelessness may be a reaction to his difficulties in real life. A bereavement, a great disappointment, separation from a loved person, great misfortunes may cause the patient to give up the struggle and to prefer death. The suicidal attempt in a way represents a call for help. The hospital and the nurse may be in a position to provide help if the urgency is clearly understood.

Occasionally the patient's suicidal attempt itself results in a solution of his problems. Relatives may become aware of his difficulties and rally round. Husband, children, parents may become more sympathetic and understanding when they realise how serious the patient's condition is. More often, particularly when the cause for the depression lies within the patient himself, admission to hospital does not make the patient feel better. His wish to die continues and makes nursing difficult. He may repeat suicidal attempts and great vigilance is required. Or he may simply not accept the nursing care he is offered and may lack the will to recover. It requires special skill to convey to a depressed patient the conviction that his life is precious, that he matters and that people care about him. The first step towards achieving this is for the nurse to recognise the problems confronting both the patient and herself. The patient's unresponsive attitude should not obscure the fact that a definite effort must be made to give genuine emotional support.

Psychiatric Consultation

Many hospitals have psychiatric out-patient clinics. The nurse's work there differs greatly from her usual duties in out-patient departments. Patients' interviews with psychiatrists are private and confidential and, except for the physical examination, the nurse is not usually present when the patient is seen. Her support is needed while the patient is waiting, or while his relatives are being interviewed, or on those occasions when the patient's anxiety is so great that he cannot wait for his next appointment, or when he has missed an interview and comes to the department later when he is not expected. The nurse has an opportunity to talk to the patient before and after the interviews and to provide the doctor with much information about his behaviour and attitude. She gets to know the patient well enough to become aware of what particular approach is likely to be reassuring. She observes changes in him which indicate his improvement or relapse and she needs skill to control him when his anxiety becomes too great.

Emotionally disturbed patients need emotional care as well as physical help. The nurse cannot prevent her own feelings from being aroused by the patient. Sometimes her feelings are uncomfortable because they may relate to some problem the nurse herself has not yet fully understood. Thoughts about death or suicide and problems related to marriage or to family tensions may arouse uncomfortable feelings. Sometimes the nurse feels uncomfortable because hostile feelings to the patient have been aroused. In her training she has learnt to like patients and feel sympathetic. Dislike of patients or anger appears wrong and she may find these hard to accept. In the presence of psychiatrically disturbed patients it is inevitable that such feelings should arise. When the nurse has learnt to accept them and to recognise her feelings rather than deny them she can begin to control them and to use her entire personality to support the patient.

SUGGESTIONS FOR FURTHER READING

ALTSCHUL, A. *Psychiatric Nursing*. 4th ed. London: Baillière Tindall, 1973.

BARNES, E. (Ed.). *Psycho-Social Nursing*. London: Tavistock, 1968.

ROBINSON, L. *Psychological Aspects of the Care of Hospitalized Patients*. Philadelphia: Davis, 1968.

STENGEL, E. *Suicide and Attempted Suicide*. Harmondsworth: Penguin, 1973.

WEDDELL, D. *Psychology applied to Nursing*. Nursing Times, 1955.

13. CHILDREN IN HOSPITAL

Separation of Young Children from Mother

In recent years much attention has been given to the experiences of small children while in hospital. There is a widespread belief that great harm can be done, not only at the time, but in the child's subsequent development if the child's basic psychological needs are not recognised.

Very small children who have not yet developed any understanding of the world around them have one overriding need: the security of the love and presence of their mother or the person who is a substitute for her. Up to the age of about $1\frac{1}{2}$ to 2 years, some believe even up to 4 years, the child cannot bear to be separated from his mother for long, least of all when new, unusual and perhaps unpleasant things are happening to him. As he is constantly learning new things he can cope with the new experience of sickness, even hospitalisation, provided he is with his mother.

In recent years this fact has been stressed to such an extent that some people believe it has been overstated. They consider that perhaps damage is not as deep or permanent as Dr Bowlby, for example, has led us to believe and that excessive emphasis on the danger of separation leads to guilt feelings in the mothers who have had to leave their babies in nurseries or hospitals, guilt feelings which are not good for the child's relationship with his mother either.

However this may be there is strong evidence that very small children suffer from a sense of loss, mourning and grief when away from their mothers. It is as if they felt that the mother must have rejected, forgotten or lost them. At first they may be tearful or angry, later there is a stage of resignation with a lack of interest and an inability to accept love or return affection. How much this affects the child's development and his ability to form relationships with other people later, depends on the duration of the separation from his mother and on the mother-child relationship before separation. Nearly always, however, the child's rate of progress, both physically and mentally, is retarded when there is a separation from his mother. On returning home the child may refuse to recognise her, may remain detached and irresponsive for some time and often revert to earlier forms of behaviour. Bowel or bladder control, for example, which may already have been achieved may again be lost, there may be nose-picking, thumb-sucking or other indications of emotional disturbance.

In Hospital with Mother

Many hospitals now make arrangements for very young babies to be admitted with their mothers if hospitalisation cannot be avoided. Contrary to fears expressed by hospital staff admission to hospital with the mother has not increased the incidence of infection. Small infants respond better to treatment if their mothers attend to their basic needs.

Older children can bear separation from their mothers more easily but their security is still dependent on the knowledge that their mothers are available and frequent visiting is important.

When a mother is admitted to hospital with her child she feels relieved to be able to carry out all those nursing measures she normally gives him. It is comforting to both mother and child if the mother can feed and wash her baby, play with him, hug and hold him whenever he is upset, tuck him in at night. The child's routine is not altered and the mother feels useful and appreciates the fact that she is fully in touch with the child's progress.

Any setbacks of course are most upsetting to the mother

and she may become very anxious if she sees her child suffer. She would, however, feel equally worried about him were she at home, unable to get adequate information. If the mother is in hospital the doctor and nursing staff can help her to express her worries, to feel secure in the knowledge that the child is having good nursing care. Her contact with other mothers, too, and the fact of being useful to the hospital are a great help.

Visiting Children in Hospital

If it is impossible for the mother to be admitted to hospital, unrestricted visiting is the next best thing. The more frequently mother comes, the less disturbing her departure becomes. Her repeated absences and reappearances are taken for granted. Most hospitals which have tried to allow unrestricted visiting have not found that the mother's presence interferes with the work. On the contrary, the help mothers can give, especially at meal times and bedtime, gives more time for the nursing of those children who are very ill or who are not visited.

Small children who are admitted to hospital may need the comfort of some tangible reminder of home. A teddy bear or a favourite piece of ribbon or cloth taken to bed with him may establish a link with his previous experience during his mother's absence. His own personal baby language and signs for toilet should be used by the hospital staff. Information about details of the child's life should be available.

The Nurse as Mother-substitute

If it is impossible for the mother to be present the nurse must attempt as far as possible to replace her. Ideally, one nurse should look after the child throughout his stay, but, as this is obviously impossible, the fewest possible number of nurses should share in his care. It is very bewildering for the child to have a large number of strangers handling him, each giving a small part of the total care. However kind the nurses are the child cannot establish emotional bonds with too many people. He needs one person who is his special nurse. Fear of showing favouritism sometimes deters nurses from singling out a particular child for attention. There is no danger of favouritism for small children unless one child were everybody's favourite, which is as impersonal a relationship as being no one's favourite. Each small child must feel he belongs to someone. If his mother has temporarily deserted him someone else, the nurse for example, must take her place.

Hospitals are sometimes afraid of the adverse effect on the child when his favourite nurse has to leave. This is, of course, a bad thing, but better than if no favourite nurse had ever existed. It is easier for a child to form a new relationship if his previous experiences have been satisfying, just as it is easier for the child to form a satisfactory relationship with the nurse if he is secure in his relationship with his mother. If nurses are assigned to the care of individual children they are in a much better position to notice signs of distress early and to respond to the child's need for comfort and companionship. If too many nurses are sharing the care of the child each may believe, from the fleeting glimpse she has, that the child has settled and is happy.

There is inevitably some disturbance when visitors leave and fear of children's tears has, in the past, led to restrictions on visiting by parents. It seems, though, as if tears and a show of emotion are much to be preferred to the restrained, detached behaviour of those children who appear to have settled down in hospital.

One of the greatest difficulties of the small child is his inability to understand the concept of time. He cannot measure the interval between his mother's visits and so he needs to be kept informed about her actions throughout the day. The nurse can give a running commentary to the child of what his mother is probably doing. 'She is cooking the dinner now for your brother, she is mending daddy's socks, she has gone out to do the shopping.' These remarks help the child to realise that life has not changed much at home. The future is measured in all the activities the child will carry out before his mother's return; for example, 'you will have your lunch, then you'll have a sleep, then the doctor will come, then we shall play, then your mummy will arrive.' Some of the hospital events can be rehearsed in play before the child's admission or before a specific treatment is carried out.

The period in hospital is not the time for a child to give up well-established habits however deplorable the nurse may think they are. Some children suck dummies when they are upset, some are fussy about food, some make a noise when they are being washed. There is no point at all in nurses being critical of the child's upbringing and in trying to change behaviour of which the mother does not disapprove. When this is attempted, the child may conform to the nurse's request during his mother's absence. When she comes, however, the conflict between nurse and parent results in more pronounced disturbance in the child and an increasingly critical attitude between parents and nurses.

Older Children in Hospital

Older children, once they have recovered from the most acute phase of the illness, enjoy the companionship in the ward. They may benefit from the independence from parental control, from the fact that nurses represent an impartial authority. Freedom from the pressures of the educational system and being the centre of attention owing to illness may contribute to a constructive use of hospital experience during development. Some children derive great benefit from the individual attention a school teacher is able to give and return to school later with enhanced prestige of having been in hospital and increased attainment. Children who do not like school benefit particularly from individual tuition.

It is important that children's routine in hospital should resemble normal life as far as possible. In order to achieve this nurses should know enough about the stages of child development to recognise whether a child's speech, play, interests and general behaviour are normal for his age or not. During illness a certain amount of regression may well occur, as it does with all patients. The fact that the child behaves in a manner more appropriate to a younger age needs to be recognised, but the child needs encouragement and help to return to more mature behaviour. He should not be penalised, for example, for wetting the bed, or for whimpering or for resorting to baby talk. But he should not be insulted by being given play material which he has outgrown, or by being placed in a cot when he is already used to a bed, or by being given a spoon to eat with when he already uses a knife and fork. A child's day normally follows a very well-established routine. There is, in the child's opinion, a right time for play, for stories, for bath and for rest. There is a time for attention from mother and a time for watching TV and a time for quiet occupation. Older children have a regular time set aside for school and work and they use for play any spare time they can find. In hospital the routine tends to be upset. Children have more time to play, sometimes more things to play with, but they may find it difficult to become interested in play when they are in strange surroundings and when play becomes the main occupation rather than the change from other events. Children's conversation is concerned with the events of daily life. They comment on all they see and do and their talk makes them more interested in what they do. If children in hospital do not have enough to do they cannot find much to talk about, and if they have no one to talk to about their play this becomes boring.

To the small child in hospital play may be of additional significance because, unlike an adult, he may be unable to explain his needs or express his feelings in words. In play he may be able to express frustration by projecting feelings on to dolls, to play out the drama of his own life in the dolls' house or to control his emotions through aggressive play. In his choice of play material he can demonstrate his level of maturity and his temporary state of regression. Such play can have therapeutic value only if it is planned and progressive. This means that the child needs time set aside regularly and a person who can devote her entire attention to him, who can enter his world and share with him the experiences of life in the ward and the memory of play that has gone before. Nurses can learn to use play therapeutically, but they are often too pressed to accord play the priority it deserves. For this reason some hospitals employ 'play ladies' who are trained to help the child and interpret his play. Communication between 'play ladies' and nurses can be of great benefit.

Discharge from Hospital

One of the dangers of long illness in childhood lies in the fact that the child may have difficulty in settling down at home. A few months in the life of a small child is a very long time. A child's development is closely linked with people and things in his environment. While in hospital he is learning about things which are not of great use to him outside. Social conventions, language, routine are totally different from the child's family culture. Meanwhile people at home change, develop new interests, start on ventures of which the child remains ignorant. When he gets back home he returns to an unfamiliar world, to an environment in which he is a stranger. He has not learnt any of the relationships he should have developed with members of his family. During his illness he is the focus of all attention. Whenever he sees his family they are all concerned with his welfare. On his return home he finds people concerned with each other, interested in the welfare of others rather than in himself. Once he is well there are no special favours, no allowance made for bad behaviour. He is expected to fit in with a way of life which is quite unfamiliar to him. It is important to remember that he needs extra love, care and attention on returning home.

It is a difficult task to help a child to use his period of sickness constructively. He must be helped to realise that there is a greater advantage in being well than in being sick. It is easy for a child to learn how to use sickness as a means of tyrannising over others and of gaining attention and affection. It takes firmness and much love and patience to give affection without waiting for the child to demand it and to treat sickness in the detached manner which makes it not worth while. Small children do not understand the meaning of sickness very clearly. They cannot understand cause and effect, symptoms and treatment. They may appear to blame the nurse or the doctor for their pain. It may be necessary to separate the functions of the nurses so that the nurse who gives the child his daily care is never associated with causing him pain. Some children appear to associate the nurse's uniform with the unpleasant experience of sickness and pain.

The child's early experiences with sickness, pain, hospitalisation, separation from his mother and being cared for by nurses may influence attitudes to sickness later in life.

SUGGESTIONS FOR FURTHER READING

BOWLBY, J. *Attachment and Loss.* Harmondsworth: Penguin, 1969.

BOWLBY, J. *Child Care and the Growth of Love.* 2nd ed. Harmondsworth: Penguin, 1965.

GOULD, J. (Ed.). *Prevention of Damaging Stress in Children.* London: Churchill, 1968.

HAWTHORN, P. J. *Nurse—I Want My Mummy*. London: Royal College of Nursing, 1974.

ROBERTSON, J. *Young Children in Hospital*. London: Tavistock, 1970.

RUTTER, M. *Maternal Deprivation Reassessed*. Harmondsworth: Penguin, 1972.

WOLFF, S. *Children under Stress*. Harmondsworth: Penguin, 1973.

14. MOTIVATION

In the last few chapters progress from childhood to old age has been described but no attempt has been made to explain why people develop in the way they do. At this stage it is intended to look, briefly, at the factors involved in explaining behaviour and the changes which occur in behaviour.

Heredity and Environment

Heredity must first of all be taken into account. People are born with varying hereditary potentialities and even if environment were completely uniform for all children, their innate differences would make them experience their environment differently.

Heredity almost certainly accounts for differences in temperament; that is, in the predominant emotional tone and the speed of reaction. It may also be responsible for intelligence and possibly for tolerance to stress situations. The particular manifestations of disturbance which a person displays under stress also appear to be partly determined by heredity. We are generally more concerned with the effect of *environment* than with that of heredity. In bringing up children parents assume that they can influence development whatever may be their child's hereditary make-up. Similarly, when we treat patients in hospital we try to bring about change by influencing their environment.

When we try to find out 'why' a person behaves as he does we are searching for 'motives' for his behaviour. Motivation can be looked at in three different ways: (*a*) by looking at the person's need or emotional state *at the time*; (*b*) by looking *backwards* at the chain of events which have led up to the present state; and (*c*) by looking *forwards* to see what the person's aims are. When for example, a patient asks for a glass of water we can explain his action:

(*a*) by stating that he is thirsty. We are stating what is the patient's internal drive or need; explanation is solely in terms of the patient's own mental state at the time.

(*b*) We can describe the circumstances which have led to the patient's thirst: the fact that he has had no drink for a long time, that he has lost blood, that he is perspiring profusely and has lost fluid. This is an explanation in terms of antecedents, looking backwards.

(*c*) We can explain that he is asking for water in order to feel cooler, refreshed, or in order to keep the nurses busy. This is an explanation in terms of purpose or aim, looking forwards. This kind of explanation is often referred to as the teleological explanation.

All these forms of explanation may be useful at times. All three types can be given in answer to the question 'why'. Few people are able to recognise their own motivation when asked to account for their own behaviour. In particular, it is rarely useful to ask someone 'why' he behaved in the way he did. Motivation can be inferred, however, if one obtains replies to specific questions. For example: 'How did you feel at the time?' asks about motivation in terms of drives.

'What happened before you did it?' asks for antecedents.

'What were you trying to do?' asks for purpose.

Physiological needs, such as hunger or thirst, can provide powerful motivation for changes in behaviour. Maslow describes a hierarchy of motives and believes that the highest motives leading to 'self-actualisation' cannot come into play until man's survival needs have been taken care of. It is well to remember that for seriously ill patients deficiency of oxygen or fluid may mean that the lower needs in the hierarchy are the most urgent determiners of behaviour.

Because in health and under normal circumstances these needs are easily satisfied, social motivation is more important for most people. The need for love, security and achievement, for example, provides social motivation.

It is wise to guard against trying to explain behaviour by reference to 'faculties', a method which was once popular. If, for example, a person remembers instructions easily nothing at all is explained by saying that he 'has a good memory'. To investigate motivation for remembering we must look at interests, attitudes, ambitions and feelings of curiosity which may help him to remember. There may be a strong feeling of need for the particular information, a strong liking for the lecturer, a feeling towards other students which makes it essential to succeed at that moment. All these are emotional states which motivate behaviour.

Emotional states give rise to physiological changes such as high blood pressure, increased blood supply to the gastric mucosa or a high pulse rate. Often people do not recognise their emotional state. It is possible to be very angry yet not to be consciously aware of it. Hidden or unconscious anger can cause a person to break something, to be sarcastic or rude, or to perspire and become flushed. Blood pressure or pulse beat may be raised without any awareness of the feelings which have caused this to happen. *Unconscious* emotional motivation is a very important driving power. We like to believe that all our actions are well thought out, rational and logical, that we are in complete control of our behaviour. In fact this is not so. Our behaviour is largely dependent on our feelings and over these we are not in control. When our feelings become too strong our ability to think clearly and logically vanishes completely: we may be blind with rage or with love, paralysed with fear, made totally irresponsible by happiness. Our interests and attitudes also depend on feelings. What we pay attention to, what we accept or reject and what we remember as relevant at any one moment are all emotionally rather than rationally controlled. Often we are totally unaware of the emotional component of our behaviour, but even when we become conscious of the feelings which accompany our actions it may be difficult to trace these feelings back to the events from which they originate.

The second type of explanation tries to establish how behaviour is determined by past events. In simple experimental situations it is easy to see how behaviour is related to cause. Depriving a rat of food, for example, can be shown to be the cause of the rat learning a path through a maze to find the food. Operating on the brain of a rat can be shown to be the cause of the rat forgetting skills it had previously learnt. As soon as we begin to study more complex human behaviour we find that cause and effect are not nearly so easy to connect:

1. The effect may be delayed so that by the time it occurs the cause is forgotten. For example, a mother's absence from her child in early infancy may much later make the child reluctant to allow the mother out of his sight. By that time the early separation may have been forgotten by the mother and by the child.

2. Several events in combination may produce a particular effect; each alone might not have done so. For example, sickness and separation from his mother combined may have ill effects on the child while sickness at home may well be coped with or a holiday away from his mother may be enjoyed. Human behaviour is so complicated that we must always look for multiple causation rather than believe that one particular line of action has any one definite result.

3. It may be difficult to understand cause and effect because so much of our behaviour has unconscious motivation. As has been shown above, feelings may relate to early

events, which have been forgotten by the time we are adults yet adult actions are, to some extent, determined by childhood experiences. Our attitudes to older people may be repetitions of our attitudes to mother, father or teacher; attitudes to our colleagues may resemble attitudes to brothers and sisters. Current behaviour may be determined by past experience, which we are unable to recall without special techniques. In some forms of psychiatric treatment patients may learn to gain control over their behaviour when the link with the origin of their emotional difficulties is made clear to them.

The third method of explaining behaviour by reference to its purpose, is sometimes the most helpful to people who are in difficulties. People do not always know what they are hoping to achieve, their aim may be unconscious just as the origin of their action is unconscious. It may, for example, be obvious to other people that a child or an adult is trying to attract attention or that he is trying to look big. It may be obvious to others that a person is trying to dominate his family by behaving as if he were an invalid or that a mother's helplessness is designed to keep her children at home, yet the people who behave in this way may be unaware of the purpose of their behaviour.

While it would be tactless and useless to try to make people aware directly of the purpose of their action, it is often useful to indicate that their purpose is understood and appreciated. The nurse can, for example, say to a patient: 'I shall call every time I pass to see if you need anything' without pointing out to the patient that he seems to be calling in order to attract attention. A mother may be able to deal with her child's attempt to delay bedtime without having to say to him 'You are only asking for a glass of water because you want to stay up longer.'

Defence Mechanisms

Even people who have some insight into their unconscious mental state refuse at times to recognise the emotion in some of their reactions. They develop an ideal picture of themselves which they endeavour to keep intact. When feelings or attitudes do not fit in with their own idea of themselves they resort to a variety of defence mechanisms.

These occur in everyone to a greater or less extent. They are mentioned in order to assist recognition of the problems confronting nurses and patients in understanding themselves and each other. The most useful mechanism is 'rationalisation'. This is a process of giving a good, logical reason for one's action, leaving out the unconscious, emotional one. The rational explanation may, of course, also be true but it may be only a partial explanation of behaviour.

Parents say that they punish children for their own good when, in fact, they may be relieving their own anger. A nurse may explain that she forgot an unpleasant task because she was too busy. The fact that it is an unpleasant and not an interesting task which is forgotten shows the emotional cause of forgetting though it is also true that she is busy. A patient may explain that she could not see the doctor sooner because she had to look after her children when, in fact, she was afraid of seeing him. The reasons people give for choosing their jobs or for leaving nursing are often examples of partial rationalisation. The emotional reasons are difficult to express and often unconscious.

Another important mechanism is 'repression', a method of dealing with uncomfortable feelings by forgetting them. The term repression does not refer to the way we remove from consciousness all but the matter we are attending to at the moment. At any one moment only a very small portion of one's total knowledge is conscious. While these lines are being read nothing other than their form and content is in the reader's consciousness. Many more things could become conscious if attempts were made to make them so. We could think of acquaintances, work in the wards, poetry that has been learnt, simple arithmetical operations, or a pleasant meal. All these ideas and thoughts are readily accessible.

Many things which have been equally well learnt or have formed vivid experiences are, however, forgotten. We have practically no recollection of the events of the first few years of life and, from then onwards, memory is patchy. Even some of the more recently acquired knowledge is mysteriously forgotten. A careful analysis of the difference between those things which are remembered and those which are forgotten shows that many of the forgotten things are unpleasant and make us uncomfortable. This kind of forgetting is called repression. It is an active process, a pushing out of consciousness of those memories, and the feelings associated with them, which are hard to bear. People may forget to turn up for appointments which they did not relish in the first instance; mistakes one made in nursing patients may be forgotten, as may also any humiliating experiences suffered in childhood or, later, at work. Other people's discomfiture is often remembered while our own is forgotten.

The normal process of repression partly accounts for the fact that we remember only a very small selection of personal details. This helps us to keep our capacity to think and learn wide open. The total amount of repressed material, however, forms part of the unconscious aspect of the personality and may affect behaviour without the person being aware of his own state of mind. When emotions remain very strong but the events are not consciously linked with them the repressed material can become a hindrance to normal development. A child, for instance, may feel angry with his mother because she punished him. If he feels too guilty about his anger he may repress the whole complex situation. He forgets about his anger and also about the events which led up to it. The behaviour he shows is gentle, kind, solicitous, submissive. He may still be unconsciously angry and this is shown by accidental breaking of his mother's favourite things, or in his bedwetting or refusal of food.

Projection. This is a device we use in interpreting the environment around us according to our own personality. We see in pictures more than can really be justified objectively. Clouds, for example, can be made into faces or animals. We see stars in certain constellations representing bears or swans when, in fact, any other interpretation is equally possible. Mountain ranges are named according to the patterns that can be seen in them. Pictures, sounds and events are always perceived according to the mood of the moment. Interest and expectation determine what is noticed from among a much greater choice of observations and mood determines their interpretation.

All these ways of making events meaningful are 'projections'. More commonly, however, the term is reserved for our attempt to deal with our own shortcomings, by seeing them in others and denying them in ourselves. When we feel guilty, for example, about our dislike of another nurse we complain that she is the one who dislikes us. People who are dishonest often attribute dishonesty to others. Racial prejudice is often attributed to other people in an attempt to deny it in oneself. The fact that our own attitudes are projected onto others may in turn affect other people's behaviour. If we go on thinking for long enough that a person is unfriendly that person will become unfriendly even if she did not feel that way at first. Our suspicions are then confirmed and our behaviour justified.

Identification. Our attitude to people depends largely on the unconscious mechanism of identification. In every situation in which we believe we understand precisely how another person feels, we identify ourselves with him. When we see a film we live through the plot as if we were one of the characters, experiencing his hopes and disappointments, his happiness and pain. Different people seeing the film at the same time may identify with different people. A young girl may come away knowing exactly how the bride felt, a young man may understand the bridegroom and an older person may understand the parents' point of view. To a certain extent each person has seen the film differently.

While we grow up we learn the roles we are going to play in life by identification with people we try to emulate. Girls identify with their mother, later perhaps with their teacher, and later still perhaps with a film star. Young nurses identify with ward sisters or matrons. It may happen that a student nurse identifies rather strongly with another student nurse, who perhaps is in trouble, so that the former is unable to see the sister's point of view. There are nurses who identify so strongly with the patients that they cannot carry out treatment successfully because they share the patients' apprehension and suffering.

Substitution of one emotional outlet for another is a common way of dealing with difficulties. Emotion may be displaced from one person to another. Anger against the ward sister may be displaced onto a more junior nurse or a patient.

Sublimation occurs when one satisfies one's emotional needs by devoting one's energies to some useful purpose. The unfulfilled need to give maternal care, for example, may find gratification in the care of the sick. Some lonely people give much love and care to cats and dogs when no opportunity occurs for giving their affection to human beings.

When emotions are so powerful that they become frightening one may resort to '*denial*' of emotions. In hospital so many painful situations occur that examples of 'denial' of feeling can easily be found among patients, relatives and nurses.

Patients may be able to tolerate their anxiety about their illness or about the family they have left behind only by appearing totally calm and unconcerned, apparently unaware of the seriousness of the situation. Bereaved relatives are often unable to cry and they sometimes say that they have no feeling at all. The optimism of some dying patients and the way patients and relatives sometimes appear as if they did not wish to be given information about the adverse prognosis of an illness is a manifestation of 'denial'. Occasionally a young mother appears not to notice that her child is deformed or mentally retarded. It is sometimes suggested that nurses protect themselves from the impact of the numerous traumatic experiences of emergencies, suffering, death and sense of responsibility by developing an unfeeling, apparently callous attitude. The use of defence mechanisms is essential to the maintenance of normal equilibrium. Difficulties only occur if the defence mechanisms are inadequate to deal with anxiety or inappropriate to the situation in which they are used. When people's behaviour cannot be understood in terms of conscious, rational explanation it becomes necessary to investigate their unconscious motivations and defence mechanisms.

15. SOME THEORIES OF DEVELOPMENT

Freud

In previous chapters we have traced development from infancy to old age. At times a possible connection between early development and later personality characteristics was pointed out and in discussing motivation it was suggested that unconscious mechanisms some of which were described may be at work. Some of the ideas and concepts we have used so far are part of a general theory of personality development put forward by Freud and modified and elaborated by some of his followers. We have so far dealt only with those aspects of Freudian psychological theory which are fairly universally accepted and applicable. The fact that we are at times unaware of the motives of our actions, that there is an unconscious part of human personality, and that early childhood influences are of importance is undisputed, though there is some controversy about the precise nature of the causal relationships between childhood experience and adult personality.

In this chapter a brief outline of the main points of psychoanalytic and related psychological theories will be given. Other psychological schools are described in later chapters.

Sigmund Freud, an Austrian physician, died in England in 1939. His main interest during and on completion of his medical studies lay in the investigation of the structure and function of the nervous system and he had done some valuable work in neurophysiology and neurological disorders before he became interested in those apparently neurological disorders in which no organic lesion could be found. He spent some time in France where he was able to observe phenomena of post-hypnotic suggestion. Although the process of inducing a hypnotic state was not clearly understood the hypnotist was able to demonstrate that his subject would carry out later, at a specified time after waking, any act suggested to her by himself.

It is, for example, possible to tell a hypnotised subject that at 3 o'clock in the afternoon she will interrupt her work, leave the room, pick up an umbrella in the hall, open it, replace it and return to her former occupation. The subject is then roused from the hypnotic state and remembers nothing of what has been said to her. At precisely 3 o'clock she becomes restless and eventually carries out the activities mentioned above and returns to her previous occupation. When questioned, she cannot explain her actions and becomes uneasy, but if one insists she finds a perfectly reasonable explanation; for example: 'I thought it was getting worn out and wanted to see if I needed to buy a new one soon.' This is rationalisation but appears to the subject to be the true reason. The suggestion made to her during hypnosis is not accessible to her conscious thoughts. It is 'unconscious' but nevertheless motivates the behaviour described. It is possible under hypnosis to suggest the loss of power of a limb, to tell the subject that he will be blind or to suggest that he will fail to recognise a particular familiar person or object. On waking from the hypnotic state the subject suffers from the symptom suggested to him. He cannot explain how he developed the symptom but is strangely indifferent to it. Under subsequent hypnotic influence the symptoms are easily removed.

The purpose of the demonstrations was to study the phenomenon of hypnosis itself. Freud, however, was struck by the significance of the fact that the subjects were unconscious of the causation of their behaviour and by the similarity between some of the symptoms which could be produced and those displayed by his patients. The most important points of Freudian theory arise from these observations; namely, the discovery of the dynamic nature of the unconscious. Freud became interested in methods of bringing some of the unconscious material back into consciousness. Under hypnosis it is possible for the subject to remember more and more of his past life. In fact it is possible to relive incidents of childhood which appeared to be completely forgotten and to experience emotions as deeply as was done originally.

Freud decided not to use hypnosis and instead developed the method of 'free association' to delve into the unconscious. If the individual feels completely relaxed and allows his ideas to wander freely, without anyone imposing any criticism or restraint, and without any selection of what appears relevant, more and more memories return to consciousness.

Psychoanalysis is the term used to describe this method. Because many people feel frightened at the thought of revealing some of their most closely guarded secrets, of which even they themselves are unaware the analyst must help the subject to relax. A friendly, non-critical, persuasive attitude is necessary, complete acceptance of anything that is said and an unhurried atmosphere. Freud felt it was an advantage for the patient to lie down on a couch for complete relaxation, and to arrange the furniture so that the facial expression of the analyst could not be observed. By using this method Freud was able to discover more and more about unconscious mental mechanisms. Because he analysed people suffering from neurotic illness he first believed that some of the events recalled from the unconscious by his patients were responsible for their illness. However, analysis of normal people and discoveries about his own unconscious convinced Freud that at least some of his findings were true of all people.

During the process of free association many unpleasant, often extremely painful events are recalled. Freud believed that these had become unconscious because they had been too painful to be dealt with consciously. He used the term 'repression' to describe the process of forgetting unpleasant, painful material. Repression is not deliberate. It is an active but unconscious way of forgetting and serves the purpose of leaving the person emotionally undisturbed. At times, however, repression is incomplete. Events are forgotten but the emotion attached to them remains and interferes in daily life. Quite inappropriate emotional reactions can occur and can be sufficiently distressing to amount to neurotic symptoms. Irrational fears, excessive hostility, a general attitude of aggression, excessive submissiveness may have their origins in repressed childhood experiences. Repression occurs in everybody. The first few years of life, which are full of important and highly significant events, are almost completely forgotten by all people. Only isolated events can be recalled without the help of psychoanalysis. During analysis the subject can recall much of his first few years without any direction or suggestion from the analyst. Recalled material is usually believed to belong as far back as the second year of life.

Freud at first believed that the recollections of his patients were accurate and factual and he was very perturbed to find that so often experiences of a sensual nature were recalled. However, he later realised that some of the recollections were not based on reality but on phantasy, although they were none the less important to the individual. Children are unable to measure time with any degree of accuracy, consequently recollections of events are not always accurately timed. There is also a lack of vocabulary during childhood to describe events and experiences clearly. People talk of their early feelings as if they were related to the state of tension in their body. In recollection adult language is used to describe events to which such language did not at the time apply and for which it may be inappropriate, with the result that reference is often made to sexual experiences in childhood. Emotions are accurately recalled and are clearly recognised, but often the event to which the emotion originally referred is described in more adult form than is justified.

Freud believed that everything that is unconscious has been repressed. We repress those things which are painful and unacceptable and consequently there must be in each of us a mechanism capable of selecting what ought to be repressed. Freud tried to present his idea in the form of a model, using words which could easily be understood but did not refer to anything else. The Latin personal pronoun EGO is used to refer to that part of the personality of which the individual is usually aware, the part referred to as the 'self'. This EGO has developed, Freud said, from the ID. The third person neuter of the pronoun *it* indicates that there is something disowned and not consciously recognised as the self.

Originally, Freud said, the infant is entirely ID, entirely motivated by impulses and urges which seek pleasure in an unrestrained, sensual way. It seeks immediate gratification of its most primitive, instinctive needs. Very soon restrictions are imposed on the infant. He cannot always obtain food or comfort as soon as he wishes. Reality impinges on the ID and restrains it. Gratification must also be postponed at times because the child's mother wishes it. Her approval may depend on some curb on the gratification of instinctive desires. The child values approval and soon begins to accept as his own those standards which are first demanded by his mother. More and more the standards of behaviour of people whose approval is valued, are accepted by the child. He forms a conscience which Freud called SUPER-EGO.

Healthy adjustment means that the EGO is well developed and strong, not easily threatened by the forces of the ID or by the excessive demands of the SUPER-EGO. Whenever there is a danger to the defences of the EGO we respond with anxiety.

The defence mechanisms previously described, or in some

people neurotic symptoms, may be used to deal with strong forces from the ID or with a SUPER-EGO which is too severe.

Freud did not explain why some people have more difficulties than others in establishing a satisfactory balance between the various aspects of personality, but he did attempt to trace certain adult personality traits back to childhood experiences. In particular he maintained that there is continuity from infancy to maturity in the way in which people derive sensual and emotional satisfaction. At each stage satisfaction must be obtained before it is possible to progress to the next phase of development. Failure at any one stage to gain satisfaction results in arrested development which Freud called 'fixation', or even a return to an earlier method of gaining satisfaction, 'regression'.

Adults obtain physical, sensual satisfaction in heterosexual relationship and orgasm. Freud believed that this special form of satisfaction can be traced back to childhood. Relaxation and satisfaction in infancy is gained during feeding by sucking. This is the *oral* stage of development. Later, elimination is a profoundly satisfying activity in the *anal* phase of development. Later still, stimulation of the genital organs by masturbation has the same effect. The next stage of sexual satisfaction is the *phallic* stage. This term refers to the male sex organ, the penis, but is used for both women and men. Freud did not say that sucking and elimination are sexual activities but that the satisfaction obtained from these activities is similar to the satisfaction obtained by adults during the sexual act. These activities are remembered during analysis with the kind of feeling which in adulthood accompanies sexual ideas. He also said that the earlier phases must necessarily be passed through during the development towards adult sexuality. After the phallic stage there is a *latency* period before more mature sexual interest arises.

The mouth continues through life to have erotic significance, for example in kissing. Psychoanalysts consider that an interest in food, sucking of sweets or pipes or smoking sometimes represent a substitute for sexual gratification. The connection between elimination and sexual development is less clear in healthy people, but the amount of secrecy, shame and guilt which often accompanies thought or talk of elimation strongly supports the connection with sex. Freud drew attention to the fact that the faecal material is the first product of the infant. He presents the faeces to the mother as a gift. Withholding faeces is a way of depriving mother of the gift, it is the child's most certain way of causing anxiety and anger in the mother, the first opportunity for asserting himself and winning a victory.

Fixation at this level of development, Freud said, not only concerns sexual development but also the adult's tendency to orderliness, his attitude to money, parsimony, or even avarice in adulthood and the way in which aggression is expressed: for example obstinacy and vindictiveness are, according to Freud, related to fixation at the *anal* level of development.

Not only adult physical satisfaction has its origin in childhood but also emotional development. Mature adults are capable of special, warm, emotional relationships with members of the family; for example, husband or wife and children. The particular feeling for a person of the opposite sex and the protective, altruistic relationship with children, are characteristics of healthy adult adjustment. Some people would go so far as to say that the fulfilment of heterosexual love in procreation represents every person's greatest desire. There are, of course, some people who cannot, through force of circumstances, find fulfilment in marriage and some who choose to devote their lives to the arts, to creative work or to public service. Some of the world's greatest creations have been produced by people who gained more satisfaction from their work than from their own personal relationships. This may be considered as a higher form of development, but Freud believed that this is 'sublimation' of the emotions which should normally be experienced in love.

Adult love is, according to Freud, a goal which is reached by going through a series of emotional experiences in child-hood. The most important of these is the experience of being loved by the mother, or by a mother substitute, quite early in infancy. All children need love and protection. The idea of an 'ideal mother' is universal. A sense of deprivation is felt when mother love is absent, or if separation from the mother occurs. However, even the best and most loving mother inevitably falls short of the child's image of the ideal mother. Every mother must at times cause frustration to the child. She may fail to pick him up when he wishes it, may interrupt feeding before the child is satisfied or fail in some other way to respond to his needs. Frustration creates anger and hate in the child, directed against the very person whom he most loves and needs. The problem of love and dealing with it, of experienc-ing hate and dealing with it without overwhelming feelings of guilt, the ambivalence of feelings to the same person, all these have to be worked through in childhood before adult adjustment is reached.

Some people believe that children should be spared the unpleasant experience of meeting frustrations. They believe that Freud, having drawn attention to the child's feeling of ambivalence or aggression, advocated that children should never be thwarted in any way. There is no justification for such a belief. On the contrary, the child gains security from the knowledge that an adult, not he himself, is in command. But he does experience strong emotions in response to frustration and may learn to deal more adequately with these emotions, if he is allowed to recognise and control them, than if he is made to repress them in order to avoid guilt feelings about them.

Adult attitudes to women, particularly to older and maternal women, may depend on the way in which feelings towards the mother are dealt with. Early in infancy the presence of the father may be felt as a threat and may often be resented because he seems to distract the mother's attention from the child. The relationship between mother, father and child provides the first opportunity for feelings of jealousy. This situation is referred to as the 'Œdipus' situation by Freud, who draws an analogy between this and the Greek story of Œdipus who, in accordance with the oracle and in spite of all precautions taken against its fulfilment, kills his father and marries his mother in ignorance of their incestuous relationship. Themes similar to that of the Œdipus saga occur in the stories of many cultures and Freud saw in this an indication of the universality of incestuous wishes in human beings. Normally, Freud thought, the Œdipus situation is resolved by identification with the parent of the child's own sex; one becoming like his father to retain his mother's love, another like her mother in order to share in the love of her father. The successful solution of the Œdipus situation results in a healthy attitude to men and women. Fixation at this stage of development may mean that excessive dependence on the mother or on a mother figure and a resentment of men is carried into adulthood—a form of maladjustment termed the 'Œdipus complex'.

In many families the father represents authority. Adult attitudes to people in authority or to those who are potentially in authority are largely patterned on attitude towards the father, though this may differ with the position fathers hold in varying cultures. Love and respect for the father may lead to an acceptance of reasonable authority and, in turn, to the use of authority in a similar manner. Resentment of the father, or the belief that the father is excessively restrictive, may lead to fear and rebellion in the face of authority and to an authoritarian attitude when the occasion arises.

Other children in the family provide an opportunity for competition, rivalry and co-operation. Freud does not say much about the effect of sibling rivalry on social development. This is discussed much more fully by Adler, one of Freud's early collaborators. The arrival of a new baby undoubtedly creates jealousy and a feeling of insecurity which need to be resolved during childhood in order to develop independence.

When school begins relationships with people outside the family become important. Teachers, for the time being, replace parents in the position of authority. They substitute impartial, detached authority for the personal one of the parents. It becomes possible for the child to see that he is equal to others, to develop a sense of justice and to dispense with an authoritarian father figure.

Some people, however, continue to feel the need for absolute authority. When they begin to doubt the absolute wisdom of their parents they obtain support from their belief in God or in the absolute truths of scientific values.

Freud has shown that these few basic attitudes to the mother, father and siblings form the pattern for later relationships. People tend to repeat over and over again the reactions they have learnt to adopt in childhood. It almost seems as if nothing can be done to change people. The emotional tie with the mother determines later reactions to other people who play a maternal role in the life of the individual, for example a nurse. Later it affects the kind of mother one turns out to be. Absence of love in childhood may well make it difficult for a person to accept love from people who are very willing to give it and may also make it difficult for her, as a parent, to give love and security to her own child.

Resentment of the father's authority in childhood tends to

be repeated when one meets any person in authority and leads to the wielding of authority in a manner resented by others. We repeat the attitudes we have learnt in childhood throughout life without being aware of their origin and often without recognising that our attitude depends more on our own personality structure than on other people's behaviour. We describe others as authoritarian or hostile, fussy or over-solicitous without becoming aware that our own attitude to them makes us see them in that light and elicits from them the very behaviour to which we refer.

This repetition of childhood attitudes to people we meet in adult life is sometimes referred to as 'transference'. Freud first used the term to describe how his patients used him as if he were the wonderful father, the loving mother or the hated authority to which they referred. They transferred onto him emotions which properly belonged to others. A positive transference, that is, the feeling of love and trust which the patient temporarily places in the analyst, is helpful during stressful phases of analysis and acts as a strong motivation to continue the analysis. Negative transference, that is hate, anger and resentment towards the analyst, can be utilised to make the patient aware of feelings of which he may have been unconscious and to help him accept characteristics hitherto repressed. Later in analysis it becomes clear to the patient that his feelings were misplaced. His judgment of the analyst becomes free from the distortion of transferred emotions and the analysis can come to an end when the patient feels he no longer needs the analyst as a target for his feelings.

In analysis transference is part of the planned process of bringing unconscious material into consciousness. In everyday life, however, transference frequently takes place. Patients in hospital sometimes behave as if they were in love with nurses when, in fact, they invest in the nurse the love which they feel for their mother. Relatives may be afraid to ask doctors for their opinion and may treat doctors with the deference which might have been appropriate for their own father. Parents often transfer to their children's teachers the mixture of fear and respect they formerly had for their own headmaster. Nurses may find that their attitude to ward sister or matron is irrational and represents a transference of feelings from their own family experience.

Transference is often very useful. In new situations and when meeting new people it is helpful to be able to use well-tried patterns of behaviour and to proceed on the assumption that the old approach will be found useful again. It helps the patient trust each nurse as if she were his mother. Order in society is more easily maintained if people respect authority automatically just as they used to do in childhood. Transference is a hindrance, however, either if the original attitudes are in themselves abnormal or if they are maladaptive to the present situation. Excessive resentfulness of authority or an excessive need for love may prevent the formation of satisfactory adult relationships. Transference also interferes with getting to know people as they really are, because the individual may go on treating them as if they possessed the characteristics which he has projected onto them.

Freud's apparently fatalistic outlook in pointing out that we cannot help behaving as we do because we merely repeat what we have learnt has, in reality, led to the awareness that change is possible, provided that people recognise the unconscious mechanisms at work in themselves as well as in other people. In psychoanalysis the analyst helps the patient to re-examine his own attitudes and, in being traced back to childhood, they automatically change. This process of re-examining attitudes can be carried out—though perhaps less thoroughly and less systematically—by anyone who is interested in human re-lationships. Nurses may find their attitudes changing con-siderably the moment they begin to ask why the patients, their colleagues or they themselves behave in the way they do.

Reports written about a patient, for example, often reveal more about the nurse's attitude than about the patient's condition. The nurse may find a particular patient irritating and trying. When she begins to investigate either what part she herself plays in provoking the patient, or what it is about herself which makes her react to this particular patient with irritation, the feeling is often recognised as transference and it then becomes possible to give the patient the care he needs without emotional interference.

Freud found that during the process of free association people began to talk of their dreams and that dreams became more frequent as analysis progressed. He began to investigate dreams and came to the conclusion that some unconscious forces are expressed in dreams. He referred to the story which is remembered as the 'manifest' content. Behind this is the 'latent' dream content; the meaning of the dream is expressed symbolically in the manifest dream content. During the dream the dreamer understands the symbolism and often wakes feeling happy and elated. When the sleeper awakes the dream appears meaningless and he wonders how the absurd dream content could ever have been thought of. Freud said the 'censor' keeps the latent dream content unconscious and even during sleep only allows disguised symbolic expression of the unconscious wishes. To understand a dream it is necessary to see what association each of the items brings forth. The symbolism used by each person is private and individual, but certain characteristics can be observed in the dreams of many people. Sometimes concrete objects represent figures of speech. We talk, for example, of feeling fenced in or of reaching rock bottom. In the dream fences or rocks may appear to represent these feelings. Often several separate parts of the dream produce the same association, this is called 'over-determination'; at other times one thing in the dream stands for a number of different ideas, referred to as 'condensation'. Some dream symbols are thought to have a sexual meaning and some occur so frequently that it is almost possible to guess at their meaning instead of inviting the dreamer to produce his own associations in order to interpret the dream. However, another person's dream cannot be accurately interpreted this way.

Freud believed that all dreams express the fulfilment of an unconscious wish. Other psychologists do not entirely agree with this statement, but they do consider that dreams are important and significant expressions of the unconscious.

Psychoanalysis is both a method of investigating personality development and a theory of personality structure. The method used by Freud has resulted in a far-reaching extension of our knowledge of human personality. It continues to be a valuable method of investigation and represents a useful preparation for those who need to know themselves better in order to learn how to understand their patients. As a method of treatment it has undergone many modifications. Some of these make treatment more acceptable to the patients and some are reputed to speed treatment. Occasionally a psychoanalytic method without modification is used in the treatment of some form of mental disorder, but this is usually too long and costly to be of practical value. Many people doubt whether, in fact, it is possible to cure mental illness by this method.

The psychoanalytic theory as developed by Freud has aroused a great deal of anger and criticism. Freudians say that the degree of 'irrational' emotion with which criticism is expressed indicates how accurate the theory is. One is profoundly uncomfortable when one is told that one is not entirely aware of one's own personality and when one's unconscious tendencies are brought out in the open. Everybody dislikes the thought of his own irrational motivation and tends to react by rejecting and denying it.

At present more objective criticism is being made by those psychologists who attempt to carry out scientifically conducted experiments to test the separate facets of the theory. There appears to be no doubt that some of the prolific hypotheses put forward by Freud will be confirmed. Much of the original criticism of Freud's theories is connected with his use of the concept of sex. Many people find it unacceptable to associate sexual concepts with child development and Freud's description of infantile sexuality has offended some people. Some of Freud's disciples have now re-examined and modified much of his theory. Less emphasis is placed on the instinctual explanations of behaviour and much more on the influence of culture.

Many people doubt some of Freud's theories because the method he used is unscientific. Usually it is only possible for anyone to practise psychoanalysis after he has himself had a personal analysis, a procedure which leads to bias by those who are analysts and excludes from discussion all those who are not.

One of the difficulties in using the psychoanalytic theory lies in the fact that it does not explain adequately how the differences in personality development occur. Freud at first believed that the traumatic events which his patients uncovered in analysis accounted for their neurotic symptoms. Later, however, he showed that even normal people recalled the same kind of childhood events. His theory reveals more of the universal patterns of development than of the causation of psychological disorder. It is also argued against the Freudian theory that many examples can be found where the same event causes diametrically opposed behaviour. The restrictions which parents impose on the child may, for example, cause hostility in later life or may result in reaction formation leaving the child too submissive and passive.

There has been some anxiety about the effect of Freud's 'deterministic' theory on the moral standards of people. If it is true that adult behaviour is caused by what happened in childhood then people cannot be held responsible for their actions. This fatalistic outlook is uncomfortable and, it is thought, could have detrimental effects on standards of behaviour. However, one's understanding of other people is helped if it is assumed that they cannot always be held responsible for their actions and opinions. Interest replaces irritation and anger. Very often it pays the student to examine his own preconceptions and prejudices and to try to bring into consciousness hidden parts of his own personality. People appear capable of guiding their own behaviour, however, they have to believe in their free will and the power to control their own actions, even when they make allowances for other people's behaviour.

The main findings of Freud are unchallenged by his collaborators and pupils. However, some deviations from his theory and elaborations of parts of the theory have occurred during the last fifty years.

In this chapter some of the main points of difference between Freud and other psychologists of the schools of *depth psychology* will be outlined. If only a few names are mentioned and less space is devoted to them than to Freud it is not because these theories are less important but because they also are based on psychoanalytic theory.

Alfred Adler

Alfred Adler, an early collaborator of Freud and one of his compatriots, later became interested, not so much in the causation and determination of behaviour, but rather in its purpose. Though he agreed with much of what Freud said about the early influence of environment Adler was primarily interested in the possibility of change. Environment and heredity, he agreed, are important, but it would be an error to believe that adult personality was entirely determined by early environment and heredity. On the contrary, we shape our experiences in the environment in which we live as a result of our own potentiality. His emphasis on the wholeness of the human organism is one of the most important contributions to current psychological thinking though his is not the only influence in this direction.

Adler's psychology can be termed 'teleological' or purposive psychology. Our main purpose in life, he said, was the effort to become powerful. We are all born helpless and in the process of growing up we aim to become strong and independent. How we do this depends partly on our view and understanding of our own inferiority, partly on the method we use to establish our strength.

The 'striving for power' arising from our 'inferiority complex' is the foundation stone on which Adlerian theory is built. Adler succeeded in explaining almost every kind of behaviour on the basis of this. Some people feel that this is an over-simplified concept of development.

The task of the child is to explore his environment, to organise his experience into a meaningful whole. Very soon everything the child sees, hears and feels and his every experience is utilised in the light of the 'scheme' which the child has already formed. He approaches new experiences with certain expectations and in the first few years develops a 'style of life' which makes his behaviour characteristic of him. Adler assumed—without examining his assumption in any critical way—that a certain style of life is good and desirable, others maladjusted and unhealthy. He believed that people ought to develop 'co-operation' and 'independence' and that it is wrong to make use of others by being helpless or excessively aggressive.

Adler was particularly interested in education and was a pioneer of child guidance. The function of the teacher or the doctor, who tries to help the child and his family, is to discover the child's particular style of life and to make the family conscious of it. The style of life can be changed by a co-operative effort of the family or the school and the child.

One of the causes of the child's original feeling of inferiority is to be found not only in his total helplessness, but in specific organic debilities. Most people are born with some organs more developed than others: they may have defective sight or hearing, a limb may be weak, speech may be impaired, ugliness, variations from the normal in height or weight may be experienced as signs of inferiority, so may sexual differences, a point on which Adler agreed with Freud. While Freud, however, talked of 'castration fears', the anxiety of the boy that he may lose his male organ and of the girl that she may have lost something she ought to have, Adler talked of the 'masculine protest'—a type of behaviour which leads to increasing competition for power.

The inferior organ is used in an attempt to become powerful. Some people compensate by greater practice and determination to develop the inferior organ. Others develop different skills and make up for deficiencies. Yet others use their deficiency to gain power over others by a show of helplessness. Organs 'speak' before real speech is developed and 'organ language' should be learnt by those who want to influence the child's development. One source of the feeling of inferiority is found in the way in which a child reacts to his position in the family. The eldest child, for example, suffers 'dethronement' when the next child is born. He feels less important, less well loved than the younger child. His way of becoming powerful may well consist in developing into a trustworthy, authoritarian type of person, adopting for himself the role of parent substitute.

Eldest children, Adler believed, often have great respect for tradition. Their outlook tends to be pessimistic and they look on the past with regret. The second child may become ambitious, optimistic, forward looking. He may be preoccupied with the need to compete and to catch up with the older child. If he cannot hope to beat the eldest in direct competition he may strike out into new fields. The youngest child, who is often petted by the parents, may reach his unique position by particular graciousness. He may dream of being the best, the most useful, the hero of the family and, if he is unable to make dreams come true by using any outstanding ability, he may do so by becoming the favourite as a result of his endearing behaviour.

The only child may develop a style of life characterised by timidity. He does not develop in competition with contemporaries. Instead, the standards of adults and their ambitions for him make the world seem to be a dangerous place. He dare not disappoint by striving and failing. If he makes no attempts to strive forwards he guards against failure and retains the protection of the adult. The position in the family in Adler's view is a very important factor in developing a style of life, but this alone does not determine development. If there is a marked difference in ability between children competition may be abandoned quite early. The child who appears to lack interest and initiative may well be one who has been discouraged in competition. The child who comes from a family in which disharmony exists between parents may become concerned with maintaining his relations with his parents rather than with the other children. Those who experience neglect may think the world is hostile and may permanently fight against imaginary enemies or guard themselves against imaginary dangers.

In investigating the style of life Adler observed the behaviour of the members of the family towards each other.

While other workers in the child guidance field tried mainly to understand the child's point of view Adler saw the whole family and discussed problems openly with parents and child simultaneously.

Adler, like Freud, was interested in the paucity of recollections of the earliest time of life, but he investigated not what was forgotten but what was remembered. The earliest recollections often give an indication of the style of life. The fact that a particular incident was recalled shows what appeared important to the child at the time. The part the child himself played in the remembered incident, whether he recalls himself as being active or passive, strong or weak, successful or a failure, is an indication of his outlook on life.

Adler paid particular attention to the pattern of behaviour which makes use of helplessness. The most powerful weapon of all is for the individual to demonstrate weakness. The weak succeed in holding back others, gaining attention, impressing everyone with the immense difficulty of their tasks. Weakness provides people with excuses for possible failure and at the same time magnifies success should it occur.

Adler's own method consisted in showing the child how successful his manoeuvres were. By making the child conscious of his effect on his parents when, for example, he is sick in the morning before going to school, the behaviour can be maintained only deliberately instead of unconsciously. He is more likely to develop a new style of life if he can be shown that power and success are to be gained by more co-operative methods. There is no danger, Adler said, in interpreting to the child what the purpose of his behaviour appears to be. If his interpretation is wrong it is rejected; if it is right it clearly strikes home whether admitted or not.

Adler's general ethical and practical outlook, his description of the tasks of life as 'communal living, work and sex', into which, he maintained, all our activities could be classified and his discussion on the meaningfulness of life have made his psychology important.

The Neo-Freudians

Many psychologists who base their work on the theories of Freud have, in their own work, placed greater emphasis on social and cultural factors than on biological ones.

The work of some anthropologists consisted in testing psychoanalytical hypotheses in the very different and more simple cultural environments of primitive societies. An advantage of the anthropological approach lies in the fact that the culture patterns are relatively fixed, social pressures are uniform on all individuals and can more easily be taken into account because of their fairly stable pattern.

Malinowski, Linton, Kardiner and *Mead* have confirmed some of the findings of psychoanalysts; on the other hand, they have shown that some assumptions which we are inclined to make about the universality of human behaviour are illfounded. There are, for example, societies in which the men manifest what we should consider feminine behaviour and vice versa. Methods of child rearing, breast feeding, weaning and toilet training vary considerably and it is not possible to be as dogmatic as formerly about the long-term influence on personality development of each method.

In the United States psychoanalytically orientated psychologists have investigated whether Freud's theory, which was developed in central Europe, applies to American culture. It would appear that in the less paternalistic society authority is less associated with the father figure than Freud believed. Maladjustment and neurotic personality traits appear to the American to be more related to the individual's position in society than to his instinctive drives.

The psychologists who have tried to develop psycho-analytic theory further are called 'Neo-Freudians'.

Horney, for example, classified people into those who move 'with', 'away from', or 'against' society. *Fromm* has examined the concept of freedom and independence as the goal of personality development. *Harry Stack Sullivan* has stressed the importance of interpersonal relationships in personality development.

In England, psychoanalysts have devoted more time to the study of social groups. Psychoanalytic theory and technique have been applied to the study of industrial problems and of social behaviour in school and work. Relationships among hospital staff, and between staff and patients, are being studied by psychologists at the Tavistock Institute of Human Relations.

Psychoanalytic theory has been taken a step further by *Melanie Klein*, working in England, who has developed techniques of psychoanalysis to be applied to young children. Her findings about phantasies and emotional development in the first few months of life make it possible to compare these with the behaviour of patients suffering from psychotic disorders, for example depression and schizophrenia, which had not previously been studied by analysts.

Mention has already been made of *Erikson*, a later psycho-analyst, whose contribution to the understanding of children and of adult personality has been considerable.

Erikson describes the stages of development as a progression of psychosocial events, the outcome of which is determined by the manner in which the person solves the special problems created by his state of maturation. Erikson lists eight stages of development. The first four of these coincide chrono-logically with Freud's stages of psychosexual development of the child, but Erikson emphasises the personality characteristics which result from the favourable or unfavourable outcome of the child's management of its developmental task. In the first years of life the child's task is to cope with dependency and to develop trust. Mistrust becomes an enduring personality characteristic if the task is not mastered.

In the second year, as the child becomes capable of independent action, success results in the development of autonomy, failure results in the development of shame and doubt.

In the third year of life when the child's phantasy life is most active and when distinction between phantasy and reality has to be mastered, the child's task is to develop initiative, but repeated failure will lead to tremendous feelings of guilt.

The child enjoys the awareness of being the cause of events but can easily feel overwhelmed if it believes itself to have caused disasters for which, in reality, it may be in no way responsible. The break up of the family for example, through a parent's death or the fact that one parent leaves the home and a divorce takes place, may result in the child blaming himself and developing guilt feelings of immense proportions.

The period which Freud describes as the 'latency period' is in Erikson's terminology, the time when the child develops 'industry' or, failing that, begins to suffer from a sense of 'inferiority'.

Freud pays relatively little attention to the development of personality after early childhood. Erikson, however, goes much more deeply into the critical experiences of adolescence and adulthood. He agrees with Freud that little boys and little girls have developed an idea of their own sex during the early phase of the oedipal situation. Adolescence is, however, the period in which 'identification' occurs with the sexual role one is later to play in life. The young boy is no longer concerned with what is expected of him as a male child, he has to learn what to expect of himself as a man, a husband, a breadwinner, a father. Similarly, the girl learns to identify with her role as a woman, a wife or a mother. Erikson shows how difficulties in the adolescent's behaviour in sexual matters, in education, in the choice of career and in adaptation to social standards can be seen as manifestations of an 'identity crisis'. The successful outcome at this stage of development is 'devotion and fidelity'.

Adults, according to Erikson, go through three more stages in which they cope in turn with problems of intimacy and solidarity to develop 'affiliation and love' with 'generativity versus self-absorption', to develop the ability to care and, lastly, with what may appear to be the essential significance of human existence, the 'purpose of being'.

At this stage the adult has developed 'integrity and wisdom'. He copes with the idea of no longer being and if successful achieves 'renunciation', if unsuccessful gives way to despair.

Erikson's interpretation of the tasks of adulthood rests on his discussion of the changing radius of significant human relationships and it has much in common with the theories of disengagement we met in the discussion of old age, and with Maslow's view on motivation we mentioned in the previous chapter.

Carl Jung

Carl Jung, a Swiss psychologist, was an early collaborator of Freud. His theory soon deviated from Freud's and in his later writings he was mainly concerned with the mythological and religious aspects of human thought. His theory is termed 'Analytical Psychology'. His most important contributions to psychology concern his theory of the collective unconscious and of personality types.

He, like Freud, realised that much of the personality is unconscious and that repression takes place to protect the conscious ego from unacceptable emotions and ideas. However, Jung believed that only some, not all, of the unconscious consists of repressed material. Jung distinguished between a 'personal' unconscious, that is, our own repressed material, and a 'collective unconscious' which we have in common with all other human beings. From the collective unconscious ideas emerge into consciousness resulting in the highly individual personality pattern of each person.

Jung's procedure of reaching the unconscious is not unlike the method followed by Freud. Jung, however, went more deeply into the analysis of phantasy and dreams and found symbols of universal meaning which he called 'archetypes'.

Individuation is the process of developing a conscious ego. Only certain aspects of personality become important and well established by this process. The whole personality consists of all aspects: those which are well developed and also those of an exactly opposite nature which remain unconscious. The total personality is one which is balanced, in which there are present at the same time characteristics of opposing nature. During the early part of life the dominant personality characteristics emerge and it is possible to classify people accordingly. The most important classification, into extraverts and introverts, is widely accepted. Extraverts are people who, in the extreme form, are easily influenced by other people's opinions of them. They are aware of the effect they have on others and are sensitive to other people's expectations. Introverts, on the other hand, are self-contained, relatively unaffected by other people and unresponsive to their environment. Most people are neither extreme extraverts nor extreme introverts. One or other of these characteristics is more fully developed in the early part of life. The opposite characteristics are present in the unconscious, capable of developing later in life. Other personality characteristics which appear in the conscious ego also have their unconscious counterparts. Masculine characteristics, which Jung called 'animus', have an unconscious feminine counterpart, 'anima'. It is also possible to distinguish characteristic reaction types; for example, feeling-thinking, sensation-intuition, one of each pair is dominantly conscious with their opposites in the unconscious. Jung believed it was the task of the second half of life to develop those aspects of personality which had remained unconscious and to endeavour to achieve a well-integrated personality by one's own efforts.

Treatment of mental disorder by Jung's method does not end with analysis. Throughout treatment the analyst interprets and helps in resynthesis and integration. Jung's belief that individuation and integration represent a process which can be achieved by deliberate effort makes his psychological outlook less deterministic than Freud's.

The psychologists mentioned in this chapter are all concerned with the study of people's development over a period of time. They trace personality back into childhood and predict how, in the future, this personality will affect people and events. They see people as agents whose actions affect the environment in which they function. Their psychological theories can be described as 'dynamic schools of psychology'.

Jung's classification into personality types forms a link between the dynamic psychologists and those who study personality by other methods.

A description of other schools of psychology will be given in Parts II and III of this book.

SUGGESTIONS FOR FURTHER READING

BROWN, J. A. C. *Freud and the Post-Freudians*. Harmondsworth: Penguin, 1961. This book describes and discusses the theories of the neo-Freudians and post-Freudians.

CRICHTON-MILLER, H. *Psychoanalysis and its Derivatives*. 2nd ed. London: Oxford University Press, 1945. This book gives a very simple account of some of the theories of personality development.

ERIKSON, E. H. *Childhood and Society*. Harmondsworth: Penguin, 1965.

FROMM, E. *Fear of Freedom*. London: Routledge & Kegan Paul, 1960.

HART, B. *The Psychology of Insanity*. 5th ed. Cambridge: Cambridge University Press, 1957. The various defence mechanisms are well explained.

LOWE, G. R. *The Growth of Personality from Infancy to Old Age*. Harmondsworth: Penguin, 1972.

STAFFORD-CLARK, D. *What Freud Really Said*. Harmondsworth: Penguin, 1967.

SULLIVAN, HARRY STACK. *Conceptions of Modern Psychiatry*. Washington: William Alanson White Psychiatric Foundation, 1947.

ZANGWILL, O. L. *An Introduction to Modern Psychology*. London: Methuen, 1950. This book has a particularly good chapter on analytical theories of psychology.

Biographies of these men make fascinating reading:

JONES, E. *The Life and Work of Sigmund Freud* (edited and abridged by Lionel Trilling and Steven Marcus). Harmondsworth: Penguin, 1964.

JUNG, F. G. *Memories, Dreams, Reflection*. London: Collins, 1967.

WAY, L. *Alfred Adler*. Harmondsworth: Penguin, 1956.

FREUD, JUNG, ADLER and the other psychologists mentioned in this chapter have written interestingly on many subjects. It is worth while to read their theories in their own original works.

PART II

Psychology and the Nurse

16. INTRODUCTION

We have seen in the first part of this book how a study of the development of personality can help us to understand patients' behaviour and attitudes to illness and the reader may well have gained a little insight into her own personality at the same time.

In this section we shall examine more specifically how a knowledge of psychology can help nurses to understand more about themselves. The next few chapters are concerned with such psychological concepts as intelligence, learning, perceiving, remembering, and we shall relate these specifically to the nurse though, of course, the knowledge can be applied to the patient as well.

Much has been written about the best methods of training student nurses. In all the discussions about professional standards and qualifications a number of problems are raised though they are seldom analysed in detail.

These are:

1. Problems related to the selection of students.
2. Problems related to the assessment of nurses.
3. Problems related to learning and teaching.

In order to give the patients the best possible nursing service we need an adequate number of people who are well qualified and an adequate number of suitable candidates for training.

What makes a candidate suitable? Can suitability be detected in advance? Can good training produce good nurses even if suitability has not been obvious from the start? How can really good nursing be measured?

The next few chapters will deal briefly with some of these

points, but no definite answer to any of the questions is possible.

How psychological knowledge can be of help to the nurse in her everyday work will also be discussed.

17. INTELLIGENCE AND INTELLIGENCE TESTING

It has become very clear from the work studies carried out that there is a considerable overlap in the tasks performed by nurses of various grades. Nursing orderlies, enrolled nurses, student nurses, trained nurses all perform some of the house-keeping tasks and give some of the basic nursing care. Enrolled nurses, student nurses, trained nurses all give technical care and all are concerned with some administrative duties. This overlap of responsibilities does not, however, mean that all nursing tasks require the same amount of knowledge or that all people could be trained to equal levels of competence.

Various aspects of nursing appear to require different degrees of intelligence. The routine housekeeping tasks and perhaps some of the basic and technical nursing skills seem to be well performed by people of relatively low intelligence. Administrative tasks, supervision, teaching and all those nursing tasks which require initiative, good judgment, adaptation to different circumstances, require a much higher degree of intelligence.

It is possible to devise different schemes of training for those who choose to perform the routine nursing tasks and for those nurses who wish to devote themselves to the organisation of the work and teaching of nurses. Whether it is desirable to do so or not is at present under discussion.

State registration implies that a nurse has acquired the necessary skill and knowledge to practise nursing on her own responsibility and that she has enough understanding of the patient's needs to be able to take the responsibility for nursing care carried out under her guidance. Such proficiency can only be reached by people of high intelligence and ability. What is meant by 'high intelligence' is the subject matter of this chapter. Whatever the nature of intelligence, however, it is certain that the Health Service needs people of all levels of ability and that good nursing care can be given by people who have undergone less rigorous training than is required for State Registration. The question then arises whether people of different abilities, and ultimately reaching different levels of professional competence, are best trained together in the first instance, or whether separate and different courses should be designed, in different educational institutions, to meet the diverse demands of the entrants to nursing.

The Briggs Report suggests that people from a wide spectrum of ability should be trained together to the point at which all reach the minimal level of proficiency, and that advanced study and specialisation should follow the common basic qualification. This suggestion is in line with the tradition of British nursing, which is based on the belief that future leaders of the profession should be thoroughly familiar with the work which people carry out under their direction. It is in line with the belief in other fields, for example in the armed forces or the police, that officers should work their way up from the ranks, and it is similar to the desire of some people in industry, that the management should have come up from the shop floor. Some people, however, criticise this approach to training on a number of grounds. Firstly, they feel it to be wasteful of time for the most able. Secondly, they believe that education in mixed ability groups is frustrating, both to the most able who may get bored, and to the less able who cannot compete. Thirdly they are afraid that standards may suffer because teaching may be aimed at the average pupil, making insufficient demands on the very able.

All these objections have been voiced too in the area of general education where some advocate selective schooling, others highlight the advantages of comprehensive education.

We shall see whether the study of the concept of intelligence can help to resolve this educational problem.

We have already mentioned that Binet found children's school progress to be commensurate with their 'intelligence quotient'. From this he concluded that intelligence was an innate capacity for *learning*. Binet's tests are still in use for the testing of small children. The version now in use is one which was standardised on English-speaking children and revised by Terman and Merrill. The performance on the test improves until approximately the age of 14 to 16, remains constant for a few years and then very gradually declines. Binet's test items cover a very wide area. Many other tests have since been devised. Some of these require the ability to read and speak the language in which tests are conducted, others rely entirely on non-verbal material; for example, shapes, patterns, colour and figures.

Since it is impossible to compare mental and chronological age with each other in adults, comparison is simply made with other people who have carried out the test and the results are given in percentiles not as intelligence quotient. 50th percentile means brighter than 49 per cent, less bright than 50 per cent of all people of the same age. 95th percentile means brighter than 94 out of every 100 people.

Supposing any particular test has 60 items and each correct answer scores 1. The total score of any one subject could range from 0 to 60. In fact, of a random selection of people, more than half might score 25 to 35. On a graph the scores would be distributed as shown in Fig. 1. This kind of distribution of scores is called a 'normal distribution' or a normal curve. The range of scores which includes roughly 68 per cent of all subjects is termed the 'standard deviation from the mean'. The score which occurs most frequently is referred to as the 'mode'.

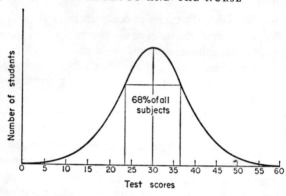

FIG. I

The normal distribution is frequently observed in the measurement of human characteristics. Height and weight are normally distributed. Examination results, too, tend to be normally distributed if the total number of candidates is large enough.

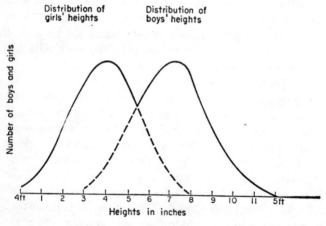

FIG. 2

Weight of men or weight of women would each be normally distributed. If the scores of men and women are put together there is a 'bimodal' curve; that is, there are two humps, as shown in Fig. 2. Whenever a bimodal distribution is discovered it means that two groups are involved rather than one: weights of boys and girls, or of Scandinavian and Chinese people, weights of nuts coming out of a bag of mixed nuts, all would show bimodal distribution.

Intelligence scores of the total population are, on the whole, normally distributed. This shows that there is a measurable characteristic common to human beings. There is no evidence of any difference between men and women or between people of different races.

At the lower end of the scale, among the people of the lowest intelligence, there is a small deviation from normal distribution suggesting that the intellectual deficiency of some people, for example those who suffered brain damage at birth or during foetal development, is different from the low intelligence of others (Fig. 3).

Tests are valid only for those people on whom they were standardised. Tests tried out on children only, for example, are

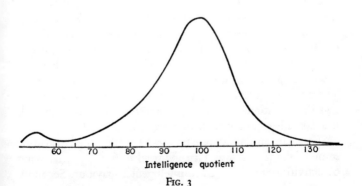

Intelligence quotient

Fig. 3

not necessarily valid for adults. To devise a test which is widely applicable it is necessary to standardise the scores on groups of children, young people, old people, town and country people, representatives of every kind of trade and profession. Standardisation means that the grading of the scores is based on a knowledge of how large numbers of people actually performed the test. A test standardised in England cannot be automatically applied, for example, in the United States of America.

A good test must be reliable and valid.

Reliability means that repeated administration will give the same result. This is like a thermometer which would be expected to show the same reading on successive occasions if circumstances had not altered.

Often with intelligence tests there is a very slight improvement after the first test; this is the result of becoming familiar with the situation and the type of information required. After the initial practice, however, no further improvement occurs if the test is reliable. For this reason some tests have a short practice test to precede them. Other tests are divided into two similar sections and one of each can be given on successive occasions.

Reliability merely means that the test score itself can be depended on. The test must, however, also be *valid*; that is, it must actually measure something real, beyond itself. It is possible to imagine a thermometer which is so reliable that it always reads 100°C.; however, it would not be valid because it would take no notice of changing conditions outside itself. There is good reason to believe that intelligence tests are valid, that there is some real quality which they measure although it is difficult to discover the nature of intelligence.

Spearman, an English psychologist, has attempted to analyse some of the tests in use. First, he tried to find out what kind of activities are involved in intelligent behaviour. Secondly he devised a method of comparing scores of various test items statistically by a method called factor analysis.

He decided that two main activities constitute intelligence:

1. The discovery of a relationship.
2. The discovery of which other factors have relationships which are similar, thereby possibly discovering new facts.

For example:

> Black is to white as Night is to . . .

The first task is to find the relationship between black and white. These are opposites. Next, find another word which has the relationship of opposite to night: the answer is *day*. This kind of activity might be called finding analogies, or forming first deductions, then inductions.

Examples of this process could be given from a wide variety of test items. For example: 1, 3, 5, 7 . . . next item 9. The relationship between these is a difference of 2; the next figure which has such a relationship to the previous figure is 9.

Another example: Pot . . . Top   Dog . . .

> These are related by reading backwards; the next word is God.

By means of mathematical calculations Spearman was led to assume that intelligence consists of a general factor, which he called 'g', and special factors called 's's. The higher the 'g' the better the performance on all types of tests and the greater the ability to learn.

The specific factors are shown by the fact that people do better in certain groups of tests than in others. For example, one person with a high general intelligence may do particularly well in all the tests involving numbers and less well in those involving words. There are special abilities of verbal facility, number sense, space, mechanical ability, musical ability, manual dexterity.

Different tests vary in the degree to which they measure 'g' and the type of 's' they are meant to measure. Usually it is wise to give a battery of tests which, between them, measure a wide variety of 's's. If only a single test is used it should, if possible, measure mainly 'g'.

Binet's test consists of such a wide variety of items that most 's' qualities are probably covered. Raven asserts that the 'g' factor in his 'Matrices' is very high. This is a test consisting of patterns and designs which are related to each other in special ways. No verbal ability is needed for this test. Raven's Progressive Matrices have been used quite extensively in student nurse selection.

On the whole, people who have a high general intelligence do better in whatever they choose to do than people with low general intelligence. It is a fallacy to believe that people who are good at Latin, for example, must be bad at sewing. They may have more special verbal ability than manual ability; but, even so, the high general intelligence will allow better performance at sewing than will be evinced by a low general intelligence with relatively high manual dexterity. In fact, however high the special ability, a low general intelligence only allows low level performance. Naturally, interest and encouragement may lead the less intelligent person to develop his skills; discouragement and lack of interest may lead the more intelligent to neglect them. But, however unfair it may seem, it is none the less true that high intelligence makes it possible to perform well all round.

There are some people, whose scores on intelligence tests are not particularly high, but who are capable of outstanding, original contributions in their sphere of interest. There are others, whose intelligence, as measured on some tests, is very high, but who perform badly on certain test items because they give solutions which are unconventional, unorthodox and not allowed for in the standardised scoring. The term 'creative intelligence' is used to describe the ability to think along original lines rather than in a manner which is convergent with the thinking of others. It is therefore possible for a person of average intelligence to obtain a very much higher score when his creative ability is measured.

In the performance of any one task there are usually more than two factors operating. Some are group factors acting over and above the specific factors. Speed, fluency, verbal facility, for example, affect any specific ability which may be shown in a test.

There is some evidence that heredity is an important factor in determining intelligence. Ability depends on the intelligence of parents and grandparents. Twins tend to resemble each other more in intelligence than other brothers and sisters resemble each other. Identical twins are more alike in intelligence than fraternal twins. The fact that identical twins raised apart are a little less alike than those brought up together shows that environment plays some part in the development of intelligence.

How big a part is played by heredity and how much intelligence is influenced by environment is at present hotly debated. Eysenck basing his writing on earlier work of A. R. Jensen has suggested that American Negroes are genetically less well endowed than American Whites. This view has come under attack from many psychologists. Some of these hold extreme views, denying the existence of innate differences of ability. They point to the fact that social class, with the accompanying educational privileges it bestows on children during the early years, is highly correlated with scores in intelligence tests, and believe that greater equality of opportunity would result in levelling up of intelligence. The more moderate critics of Eysenck's view accept that variations in ability are at least partly attributable to genetic influences but they show that the brain is susceptible to external influences and they point out that the psychologists' efforts are more profitably spent in finding methods of social and cultural enrichment to try to eliminate individual differences, than in devising selection procedures designed to perpetuate the social class differences in intellectual endowment. It is not possible to measure directly the innate aspect of intelligence. This can only be inferred from the actual performance in daily life. Hebb has suggested that one can think of innate intelligence as 'intelligence A'. This potential intelligence with which a person is endowed, cannot be measured. 'Intelligence B' is the effective intelligence measurable by tests. It is the result of modification of intelligence A by environmental influences which can start during intrauterine life and continue during the critical periods of child development.

Intelligent parents, on the whole, have more highly intelligent children than dull parents. While it would appear that heredity is involved it was noticed that some children, who changed their environment, dramatically improved in intelligence scores. Children moved from orphanages to foster homes, for example, or from bad homes to good ones, made rapid strides and showed much higher scores in later tests.

Intelligence can be developed only through training. The child who plays, who explores, who is allowed to make mistakes, to handle everything, who is constantly active, has the opportunity to develop his intelligence to the full. It is interesting to note that Piaget, who approached the investigation of the nature of intelligence from an entirely different angle, arrived at similar conclusions. He tried to describe how children's thought processes developed and showed that the child can not have a concept of an object without 'sensorimotor' organisation, that is without having the opportunity to discover for himself in active play how the various attributes of the object relate to each other. In order to play as described, he needs security, love and encouragement. Children in institutions, such as orphanages or sometimes hospitals, may lack the normal facilities and normal encouragement to learn and therefore may appear unintelligent. In extreme cases of deprivation children may, in fact, appear to be severely defective. If love, affection and security are later given and if the child has not suffered to such an extent that he has become incapable of responding, very rapid improvement in intelligence will occur.

Children who suffer from a physical handicap may also fail to develop their intelligence to the full. Poor eyesight, for example, deprives the child of much visual stimulation; deafness makes it difficult for the child to communicate and to develop speech. The spastic child, or the child who is partially paralysed, cannot play as other children do; he lacks the opportunity to develop manipulative skills or to explore his environment. The child who suffers from epilepsy cannot join in the activities of other children and may therefore be retarded.

Many highly intelligent people have few children while many less intelligent parents have large families. There could, therefore, be a fear that the general level of intelligence is declining. Reasons for the difference in size of family are obvious: longer education, higher economic demands for their family, better understanding of birth control, greater ability to control sex relationships restrict the families of some of the professional people. People of lower intelligence leave school earlier, may feel sufficiently mature at an early age to start a family. They may be more improvident and less able to practise birth control or restraint. They may not expect a high economic standard and therefore not mind having larger families. In fact, however, there is little evidence of any decline in intelligence. Although parents and children are similar in intelligence children tend to be nearer average than their parents.

Outstandingly brilliant children can be born in any family just as severely defective children can be born to very intelligent parents. Some people believe that people of subnormal intelligence should be prevented from having children. In fact, children are often much brighter than their parents, a factor which makes parenthood all the more difficult for the dull parents and means that some help must be made available to them.

It is possible for people of varying intelligence to reach similar levels of attainment, though the brighter person takes a shorter time than the less intelligent. The brighter person can do it unaided, the less intelligent may need help. This has important implications for all fields of education, not least for nursing education.

Investigations have shown that at least average intelligence is needed to pass examinations for the Registers in nursing with a fair amount of ease. Higher intelligence is needed to progress in nursing to the position of ward sister, administrative positions or tutoring and for work where no immediate supervision is available, such as public health.

It would be easy if only candidates of superior intelligence could be selected. In fact, of course, there are few people in that category and some of them are needed for teaching, research and other academic careers. For nursing, therefore, we must recruit people with sufficiently high intelligence to understand the work without setting the standards unrealistically high and without discouraging the very brightest, who are needed as potential leaders.

In our state educational system records from secondary school should be as clear a guide to intelligence as a test. People who have sufficient intelligence to cope with nurse training should have managed to obtain passes in a few subjects in the General Certificate of Education and this is required by the General Nursing Councils as the minimum educational standard. True, some children waste time at school and, though they have high intelligence, do not achieve great examination success. Intelligence tests may then be useful in selection to diagnose underachievement and to predict the likelihood of success in training.

In everyday life people of various levels of intelligence must be able to live with each other. Perhaps particularly in nursing an awareness of the difficulties of the less intelligent and a natural acceptance of the abilities of those of high intelligence are important. Student nurses of high intelligence may have to work with senior nurses whose grasp and understanding are less quick. It is often irritating to those students to find their questions brushed aside or inadequately answered. It helps the student if she can understand that the senior nurse's greater experience may enable her to show rather than tell, that she may find it difficult to express herself logically but finds it easier to teach by doing. On the other hand, senior nurses need to be aware of the abilities and limitations of the junior staff and must be able to adjust their expectations and method of instruction.

The amount of learning expected from the brighter student might have to be greater than that to be expected from the less gifted. Discouragement of the slow has to be avoided and the stimulus of competition must not be sacrificed.

Many nurses find that patients of very high intelligence tax them considerably. Patients who have superior knowledge and ability benefit if their contributions can be used constructively. Nurses need training in communication in order to feel secure with such patients. It is possible that ease of communication between people of different intelligence levels could be increased if, in training, students were not too rigidly segregated according to intelligence.

Intelligence declines with advancing years; from early adulthood very slowly, after middle age slightly more rapidly. This decline is, however, very gradual and not noticeable except on testing. The accumulation of knowledge, the wider frame of reference and the greater understanding of the more mature person may make learning easier in spite of the slight decline in intelligence. It is a fallacy to believe that nothing new can be learnt after adolescence. Obviously, too, the higher the intelligence the less handicap results from the very slow decline of middle age. A very rapid decline in intelligence occurs only when the brain is damaged, either by tumours, injury, drugs, toxins, chronic infections, alcohol, or the effects of vascular disturbances. The decline of intelligence in old age is best shown if one uses a number of intelligence tests which measure different mental skills, or if one uses a test which incorporates a number of subtests. A combination of a verbal and a performance test may, for example,

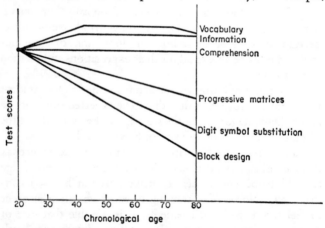

FIG. 4. Performance in certain subjects slowly deteriorates between the the age of 20 and 80.

be used. The Wechsler–Bellevue intelligence test is very suitable because of its wide range of subtests. On the subtests known as the 'Digit Symbol Substitution' and the 'Block Design Test' deterioration with age is more marked than on the other tests. In these tests speed is an important element and older people perform better if they can take as much time as they feel they need rather than feeling compelled to work fast. They also find it difficult to apply a set of specific rules or instructions to their performance. They can cope well with those tests in which previous experience can be applied.

In severe brain damage a decline in intelligence, called 'dementia', is noticeable in the behaviour and conversation of the patient and clearly measured in intelligence tests. One of the characteristics of dementia is the decline in those abilities which involve judgment, discrimination, remembering instructions. Intelligence tests can be used to exclude mental deficiency or dementia before a diagnosis is made of some other illness. In some mental disorders the patient's behaviour may be so disordered that dementia is suspected. In schizophrenia for example the patient's logic is all his own, other people find it difficult to follow his reasoning. His actions may appear to lack meaning and not to be based on ordinary good judgment. In depression the patient may be inactive, uninterested, apparently lacking understanding. Yet intelligence tests in these conditions, provided the patient can be persuaded to co-operate, will show that his intelligence is in no way impaired.

Intelligence tests often help to diagnose emotional disturbances in children. Subnormality should be diagnosed as early as possible in order to begin special training early and intelligence tests can help to find out if this is necessary. They should also be used when children's bad behaviour at school is not fully understood. Children of low intelligence may respond to the pressure of school and the parents' ambition with resentment, rebelliousness, or complete discouragement and apathy. In the education and training of mentally subnormal children it is particularly important, not only to assess the overall level of intelligence but also to investigate specific areas of relatively high and low achievement.

There is some danger that those concerned with the upbringing of mentally subnormal children may be satisfied with too low a level of achievement, assuming that low intelligence prevents the child from making further progress. Many children are unnecessarily handicapped because of the low expectation people have of them and they fail to achieve the maximum social competence of which they are capable.

Children with high intelligence may find the work too boring, cease to pay attention and then begin to do badly at school. It is always of interest to find out why children, or even some grown-up students, fail in their studies in spite of possessing superior intelligence. It may be due to emotional trouble which interferes with learning. In child guidance, student selection and occupational guidance it is important to assess how effectively the individual uses his intelligence.

SUGGESTIONS FOR FURTHER READING

BUTCHER, H. J. *Human Intelligence: Its Nature and Assessment*. London: Methuen, 1968.

GETZELS, J. W. and JACKSON, P. W. *Creativity and Intelligence*. London: Wiley, 1962.

HEBB, D. O. *The Organization of Behaviour*. London: Chapman and Hall, 1949. (Also new paperback ed. published Wiley.)

HEIM, A. *Intelligence and Personality*. Harmondsworth: Penguin, 1970.

HUDSON, L. *Contrary Imaginations*. Harmondsworth: Penguin, 1967.

RICHARDSON, K. and SEARS, D. *Race, Culture and Intelligence*. Harmondsworth: Penguin, 1972.

VERNON, P. E. *The Structure of Human Abilities*. 2nd ed. London: Methuen, 1961.

WISEMAN, S. (Ed.). *Intelligence and Ability*. Harmondsworth: Penguin, 1967.

SOME EXAMPLES TAKEN FROM
INTELLIGENCE TESTS

ANALOGIES: Underline the correct answer.

up is to *down* as *high* is to ...	Book, Sky, Low
fire is to *hot* as *ice* is to ...	Water, Solid, Cold
cause is to *effect* as *disease* is to ...	Reason, Death, Life
The day before yesterday is to *the day after tomorrow* as *Saturday* is to ...	Sunday, Monday, Wednesday

OPPOSITES: Where the words mean the same or nearly the same underline *same*, where they mean the opposite or nearly the opposite underline *opposite*.

Dry ... Wet	Same, Opposite
Dirty ... Unclean	Same, Opposite
Haughty ... Arrogant	Same, Opposite
Relinquish ... Cede	Same, Opposite
Munificent ... Parsimonious	Same, Opposite

REASONING: (*a*) Find the two letters or numbers which continue the series.

30, 50, 70, 90, ...

Z, A, Y, B, ...

$\frac{1}{4}, \frac{1}{2}, \frac{3}{4}, 1, ...$

(*b*) Underline the two words which do not belong to the same category as the rest.

Hat, Boot, Head, Shoe, Glove, Hand, Dress, Stocking.

Apple, Plum, Rose, Orange, Apricot, Cabbage, Cherry.

DIGIT SYMBOL SUBSTITUTION:

1	2	3	4
/	1°	C	+

2	1	4	3	2	4	1	3

CREATIVE INTELLIGENCE: How many uses can you suggest for:

a knitting needle, a piece of string, a brick.

CONDUCT OF INTELLIGENCE TESTS

Intelligence tests should always be administered under carefully controlled conditions. The candidate should be comfortable, instructions should be given exactly as prescribed and timing strictly adhered to.

Tests start with easy items and gradually become more difficult. Later items often follow logically from earlier ones. The subject who works systematically through a test can often solve problems which, taken out of context, may appear excessively difficult. Tests should range beyond the ability of the subjects to be tested. The candidate is therefore often told before he begins that he may not be able to complete the test in the time allowed.

18. PERSONALITY AND PERSONALITY TESTS

It is generally agreed that intelligence is not the only characteristic which determines success or failure in nursing. 'Personality' is often said to be more important than intelligence.

Psychologically speaking this statement is meaningless because intelligence is one of the aspects of personality, just as beauty, height, posture or other aspects of physical appearance are parts of personality. What is meant by this statement is that other personality characteristics should be taken into account as well as intelligence.

The study of these personality characteristics is known as 'psychometrics'. It represents an attempt to investigate 'individual differences'. First, one needs to describe the distribution of personality attributes in the population; next, one needs to specify how individuals differ from each other with respect to these attributes; thirdly one can try to find the norms of a particular occupational group or a particular section of the community.

If we try to describe desirable personality characteristics for nurses we find that many methods are used.

1. The most common way to describe the ideal nurse is to enumerate a number of qualities she should possess. Such characteristics as patience, tolerance, honesty, perseverance, conscientiousness, thoroughness, initiative are often mentioned. These are referred to as *personality traits*. A trait is a tendency to behave in a consistent manner in various situations. The knowledge that a person possesses a particular personality trait makes prediction of her behaviour possible. A nurse who is thorough, for example, carries out a variety of tasks with thoroughness. She is thorough in her studies,

in her routine ward duties, in her attempt to get to know patients, in her dealings with ward management and in her own personal affairs. If she is asked to carry out a job it can be predicted that she will do it thoroughly, whatever it may be.

Of course the question of whether a nurse has a particular trait can be answered only from observation of her behaviour; thus, to say that she is thorough simply means that she has been observed to demonstrate this trait repeatedly in the past.

Some personality traits have been carefully investigated in order to find out whether the use of a single word, describing a trait, corresponds to some unifying characteristic of personality. Honesty, for example, has been the subject of study in a large sample of children. They were given every possible opportunity to cheat and behave dishonestly in many different situations. During school work they had the opportunity to cheat by looking up the answers or by copying from others. They could cheat in their report of the results or of the time they took over individual items. They also had the opportunity to steal or to tell lies. It became obvious in these investigations that honesty or deceit were not in fact single traits. Some children cheated in their work, but not in their handling of property. Some gave false reports but worked without cheating; some told lies about their work, but not about their behaviour. Some children may cheat at school but not at home. This study was carried out by Hartshorne and May.

Most of the traits we look for in nurses have not been as carefully examined, but it is probable that they, too, are more complex than would appear. It is necessary to ask not simply whether or not a nurse possesses any given trait, but rather how much of it she has, in what circumstances she displays it and whether the trait is specific to particular circumstances or fairly generalised.

2. Another way of describing a suitable or unsuitable personality is to refer to the *emotional state* or *temperament*.

Such characteristics as moodiness, emotional instability, being easily upset are less desirable qualities. Cheerfulness and an even *temperament* are more desirable in the nurse.

Temperament is the term used to refer to the way in which emotions are expressed and experienced over a long period of time. Mood describes the emotion prevailing for a short period.

At the moment of hearing bad news, for example, a person may feel sad. This is a brief experience of an emotion. If sadness persists it is called depression, which is a mood which may last all day or several days or weeks. Some people become depressed at frequent intervals. They tend to feel happy and elated at times and then plunge into a depressive mood. This is their *temperament*; it is one of mood swings sometimes called cyclothymic.

Classification of personality according to temperament has been attempted many times. It is always recognised that temperament is in some way connected with bodily structure and particularly with the functioning of the endocrine glands. Such a description as phlegmatic implies that the calm, unemotional person has large amounts of mucous secretion, a true observation of the parasympathetic activity in a relaxed calm state. The choleric or angry, irritable person, who loses his temper frequently, was thought to have excessive secretion of bile. The sanguine person who has mood swings and shows excitement and animated passions was thought to be full-blooded.

Kretschmer associated different temperaments with body build. He thought that a schizoid temperament, a reserved, shy, withdrawn, emotionally shallow personality is most often found in asthenic people; that is, people who are long and thin in body build. Cycloid temperament, mood swings from elated to depressed and emotional lability, he associated with pyknic body build, a short and stocky physique.

Shakespeare seemed to have similar ideas; in *Julius Caesar* he says:

Let me have men about me that are fat;
Sleek-headed men, and such as sleep o' nights;
Yond Cassius has a lean and hungry look;
He thinks too much: such men are dangerous.

The American psychologist, Sheldon, describes a similar association of temperament with body structure but divides bodily types according to the development of various tissues during the growth of the foetus.

The fertilised ovum splits until a ball of cells is formed which then arranges itelf into three layers. The outer layer is called ectomorphic; the middle, metamorphic; the inner one, endomorphic. As the embryo develops the ectomorphic layer forms mainly skin and nervous system; the metamorphic layer, bones and muscle; the endomorphic layer the internal viscera. Sheldon believes that temperament is associated with the predominance of any one of these layers.

Although people's 'temperament' is often referred to there is very little to show whether any particular temperament makes one person more suited to nursing than any other temperament. People whose mood varies are sometimes difficult to get on with. Student nurses may find it a strain to have to adjust to the mood of the ward sister. The temperament of the nurse certainly has some effect on the feelings of the patient. However, it would be wrong to say that this is a bad thing. On the whole it is easier to feel strongly about people whose emotions are strong and who express their emotions. Excessive placidity may become very disconcerting.

In adjusting our behaviour we often take into account what emotional reaction it is likely to provoke in others. If other people's emotions are quite erratic it becomes difficult to take them into account; if emotional response is absent guidance is missing. Some patients assume, for example, that the nurse's mood is related to what they themselves have said or done. They are frightened at times by what appear to them to be erratic moods in nurses, but they do not find permanent cheerfulness very helpful either.

The nurse's inexplicable mood may not be a response to the patient at all, but perhaps to some other situation; for example, bad news from home, or a disagreement with the ward sister, or simply the manifestation of her emotional lability. Because the patient needs the nurse's emotional response to his own actions he interprets them as such.

It is true that some people are temperamentally more suited to nursing than others, but except in extremes it would be very difficult to select candidates according to temperament. Temperament is inclined to change somewhat with age. Adolescents are frequently moody. In middle age, probably associated with glandular changes, mood swings again frequently occur. In women this may become most troublesome at the time of the menopause; in men, rather later. Disorders of endocrine glands, for example the thyroid glands, are often accompanied by changes in temperament.

3. Another way of describing a nurse's personality consists in referring to *personality type*. There is an overlap between descriptions of temperament and type. Certain temperaments are believed to be associated with body types as already referred to.

Descriptions of a person as shy, reserved, keeping himself to himself, or, on the other hand, descriptions of hearty, easy-going people who are the life and soul of the party, good mixers, popular, are descriptions of the introvert and extravert personality types respectively. These terms were first used by Jung and introvert and extravert characteristics have been described by many psychologists.

Introverted people do not react very much to other people's feelings. Their own interests and activities are not directed towards others. Extraverts are aware of the effect they have on others and their behaviour is guided by their relationship to people. Most people are not entirely introverted or extraverted but exhibit characteristics of both types.

There is no special merit in being either introvert or extravert. Some extraverts, by their ability to respond to other people's moods, are excellent company and give valuable contributions to society. The morale and tone of a nurse's home, sometimes the atmosphere of a ward—certainly the success of a party—depends on the number of extraverts there. On the other hand extraverts are often inclined to show off, to put themselves in the limelight and to depend on other people's approval so much that they become irritating or overpowering.

Introverts sometimes make other people uncomfortable because they appear too little concerned with what is going on. On the other hand their thoughtful comment and their strong and stable emotional support, when they are able to give it, can be extremely valuable to their colleagues and to patients. Again it seems as if in nursing there is room for both types except perhaps extremes in either of them.

4. The most common way of describing desirable personality characteristics is to refer to *attitudes* and *sentiments*.

Nurses are expected to show concern for the patient's well-being, to be polite to patients and staff, loyal to the hospital, to have high moral principles, to adhere to a code of ethics laid down by the profession and to respect the knowledge of their seniors.

An attitude is an orientation towards an object or situation, a readiness to respond in a predetermined manner. Trust in a nurse, for example, is an attitude in the patient which helps him to respond to the care the nurse is proposing to give, without critical awareness and without needing proof of the nurse's ability.

Our attitudes help us to act quickly. Without attitudes to predetermine our actions we would have to examine the facts and merits of every situation before we responded to them. An attitude of obedience, for example, is desirable at times of emergency.

Attitudes are acquired during all periods of development. We have already seen how attitudes to parents may later determine attitudes to other people who are parent-like. Ward sisters, tutors or matrons are often approached with the same attitude as the mother, teacher or headmistress used to be. Patients adopt towards nurses the attitudes they learnt during childhood play. Doctors are often approached with the attitude appropriate to the father at the time when he seemed to be very big and wonderful.

Some attitudes are learnt later in life. During nurse training the student hopes to acquire useful attitudes to the hospital, staff, patients and their families, the community and her own friends. Attitudes to suffering, sickness and death are liable to undergo modification during a nursing career. Prejudice is really the same thing as an unfavourable attitude, but because prejudice is an attitude with a very strong emotional factor it is difficult to change. We talk of prejudice against racial or national groups, in religion and politics whenever we refer to tendencies to respond in a predetermined way which interferes with rational judgment. There is prejudice, too, in some people's attitude to mental disorder, or to venereal disease, to people of a certain social class, either much above or much below their own, and in attitudes to people in a position of authority or to people over whom authority must be exercised. Some general statements which are often heard that 'all nurses are wonderful', 'all sisters are dragons', 'all student nurses are lazy' are clearly evidence of prejudice.

While attitudes can be helpful in facilitating action they have the disadvantage of covering too wide a field. This is obvious in unfavourable attitudes or prejudices, but it is equally true of positive attitudes. Universal distrust, for example, is as useless as universal trust.

The infant shows the same attitude to a very large number of experiences: interest, curiosity, approach, indicate a positive attitude to people and objects; fear, withdrawal and crying, a negative attitude. Gradually the child learns to discriminate and attitudes become more specific. Some basic attitudes remain with us through life unless very special efforts are made to change them. Attitudes to such figures in our lives as our mother and father, brothers and sisters, tend to be repeated, especially in times of stress, and are characterised by a return to more childish behaviour. It is the function of training to develop and change attitudes and to help students to adopt a more discriminating approach.

Measurement of attitudes is necessary in order to define the aim of training and to measure progress, but it is unreasonable to suppose that all the right attitudes should already exist before commencement of training or even by the end of a period of training.

The term *sentiment* was formerly used in discussions about attitudes. Sentiments are emotional attitudes to particular events, objects or ideas. Love, hate, loyalty and patriotism are examples of sentiments. It is now more common to use the term 'attitudes' to include the orientation towards concepts or situations as well as the readiness to respond. If people are in love they experience a tremendously wide range of emotions which depend on their circumstances. There is elation while they are together; sadness when apart; hope, confidence, curiosity when things go well; despair, resignation, despondency when they go badly; anger towards anyone who threatens the loved person; protective feelings to the loved person.

Attitudes strongly influence a person's actions even if, at times, he is not entirely conscious of them.

In childhood attitudes to only a few people motivate behaviour. Quite strong attitudes can also exist for such objects as teddy bears, dolls and toys. Often conflicting feelings arise: love and hate for the mother and father occur at the same time. Gradually the objects towards which we have strong attitudes change and many attitudes merge and form an integrated pattern. We no longer feel strongly for dolls, but perhaps for the home, street or village, or for the part of the country in which we were born. Later the whole country or the whole nation can become the object of our attitude system. Some vestige of early sentiment often remains. It may be recognised as belonging to the past and the experience of the sentiment may become consciously pleasurable. 'Sentimentality' is the term used to describe enjoyment of sentiment. There are three important attitude systems in adults: about themselves, about other people and about abstract ideas.

It is essential to have a certain amount of self-esteem. Without it all initiative, all interest and all esteem for others vanish. To some extent this is self-love, with all the characteristics of love: pleasure in success, sadness in failure, admiration of our own ability, alternating with criticism and disgust at our own shortcomings. This regard for self is essential if an individual is to have any regard for others and also depends on the regard in which he is held by others. It is not at all incompatible with humility, self-abasement and self-criticism. All these attitudes are an indication that a person cares enough about himself to look seriously at his own actions.

Self-esteem is essential to nurses and patients alike. The nurse's function is to foster the patient's self-esteem in every possible way, remembering that sickness, helplessness and dependence tend to make him lose his self-esteem very quickly. Loss of responsibility during illness, humiliation at having lost control, the indignity of having to submit to the ministration of doctors and nurses, all tend to lower self-esteem. In mental illness particularly self-esteem is easily lost. To build it up again constitutes one of the most difficult tasks of the nurse. To be successful the nurse must have enough confidence in herself. In relationships with others a systematic building up of self-esteem is essential.

Attitudes about abstract ideas include hatred for suffering, love of service to others, love of justice, freedom and democracy. These are all-pervasive and create a value system which affects the individual's attitudes in all his work, his choice of friends and his interest in world affairs.

The strength of generalised abstract value systems varies during adult life. Often these feelings are strongest in adolescence, waning perhaps while strong feelings for particular people develop, for example during courtship, marriage and early parenthood, but growing strong again in maturity. Strong feelings about universal suffering may be a powerful motivating force in nursing. However, it is possible to give excellent nursing care to patients without experiencing this, and there are people whose very strong and genuine concern for the welfare of humanity as a whole prevents them from giving adequate thought to the detailed attention required in nursing a particular patient.

5. *Interests and aptitudes* are important personality characteristics. These are closely related to attitudes and ability. Often students are asked why they have chosen nursing. Their usual answer is that they are *interested*. The interest may be in people, or in disease, or in the theoretical study of biological sciences. Some students may find it difficult to know where exactly their interest lies, but conversation about the work itself will reveal whether they are attracted by the curriculum or by the prospect of doing practical work in the ward. Interest is essential to the acquisition of knowledge and it grows with knowledge.

Conversation about the subject in which a person claims to be interested reveals as a rule how far the interest goes. For example people interested in stamp collecting invariably know enough about the subject to maintain long conversations about it and, with every contact they make, interest grows.

Some interests develop because special skills make it possible to go more deeply into the subject than is possible for other people. Manual dexterity, for example, may perhaps be an essential skill for anyone who wishes to take his watch to pieces and develop an interest in watch repairing. Technical aptitude may be necessary for an interest in motor mechanics. Nursing requires a certain number of special aptitudes: manual dexterity is useful in practical bedside nursing and tray and trolley setting; speed is useful in all nursing tasks. Linguistic ability makes examinations easier, musical aptitude is an asset in a nurse's home life. Some special aptitudes in sports, music or art may be of the greatest value to mental nurses in the rehabilitation of patients. No one special aptitude is used all the time in nursing and, on the whole, average endowment in most respects makes training possible.

It was said at the beginning of this chapter that personality characteristics, other than intelligence, may be important in determining success or failure in nursing. If it were known what personality characteristics unsuccessful nurses share with each other, but not with successful nurses, it might become possible in future to use personality tests as part of a selection procedure for nursing posts. Research along these lines is advocated in the Briggs Report.

Methods of Measuring Personality

A *criterion* is needed by which good nurses may be measured, some agreed standard against which to measure success or failure. The first difficulty in arriving at a suitable standard is to find out whose judgment can be relied on. The same nurse may be thought excellent by the ward sister and much less so by her colleagues and the patients. The reverse is also possible in that nurses who are particularly kind, considerate and courteous to patients are criticised by senior staff for being slow and forgetting some of their work. The following are some of the ways by which a criterion for selection might be arrived at.

1. *Open Reports*

These are most widely relied on. The assumption that ward sisters know which of their students are good is, on the whole, well justified.

One method of writing reports consists in using blank paper and writing whatever appears to the writer to be important. This method will highlight the student's faults and merits and its overall tone gives an indication of the student's general ability. Details, examples and episodes may be mentioned. There are some serious drawbacks to this method. First, it is possible to leave out statements about large areas of the student's personality. This happens either deliberately about unfavourable characteristics on which the sister prefers not to report, or it may happen unwittingly about all those aspects which are unspectacular yet may be the essential ingredients of a good nurse. Another drawback is the emphasis every sister places on those aspects which to her appear to be of particular importance. One sister may always comment on tidiness and punctuality; another one never thinks of mentioning these but always refers to an ability to teach others or to co-operate. This bias about certain aspects of the work makes comparisons of successive reports difficult.

Halo effect is a further drawback of this method of reporting. Any one outstanding characteristic may influence the opinion of the reporter to such an extent that the whole report is coloured by it.

2. *Rating*

These difficulties can be overcome if the report is made in the form of a rating scale.

The reporter is not given an entirely free hand. Instead she is given a number of headings and asked to state the degree to which the characteristic is present in the student.

In an open report, for example, the sister may mention that the student is not always punctual. This may mean that she arrived late on one occasion, or, on the other hand, it may mean the student is unpunctual so often that it had to be mentioned in the report.

If the method of rating is used the question of punctuality must always be filled in because the heading already appears on the paper. The sister may be asked to rate each item on the report on a 5-point scale, meaning that;

    (i) the nurse is always punctual,
   (ii) usually punctual,
  (iii) average in punctuality,
  (iv) frequently unpunctual,
   (v) always unpunctual.

On some report forms the questions are all set out and the sister ticks the answer which applies. This makes it possible to give detailed examples of what is meant by the rating, for example:

> Her work is always accurately done without any need to supervise.
> She usually works accurately, occasionally asks for guidance.
> She works well with only cursory supervision.
> She works well only when supervised.
> She does nothing at all unless closely supervised.

This kind of reporting makes it necessary for the sister to think about every aspect of the nurse's work, even those she would otherwise have thought unimportant.

Rating will give a fairly clear picture as to whether a student is average, above or below average, or quite outstandingly good or bad.

Although this has been discussed here in relation to the personality assessment of the nurse the method of reporting under pre-set headings and with some idea of rating has much to recommend it in reporting patients' progress, and particularly on the behaviour, attitudes and interests of mentally ill patients.

3. Many requests for reports are drawn up in the form of a questionnaire and many suffer from serious shortcomings. The construction of *questionnaires* is a highly skilled task. No questionnaire should be put into use until it has been thoroughly tested. Questions are often ambiguous, they may seem to range too widely to be answered adequately, or may seem too narrow to allow for a full answer. There may be leading questions or questions allowing for too many alternatives. It is not always possible to know in advance which questions will prove relevant and which may cause so much embarrassment that their inclusion is not worth while. It is often necessary to obtain the required information by a series of questions or by an indirect approach. It may be advantageous to present a number of statements rather than questions and to ask for one of the statements to be ticked.

Systematic and careful reporting at regular intervals can give a good idea of a nurse's ability and personality. The reports will show how good she was at the beginning, how much improvement occurs as a result of training, how good she may be expected to be by the end of training. The comparison between beginning and end should be either a measure of the success of training, or should make it possible to detect which characteristics are so essential to training as to make their presence a necessary condition of selection. There are obvious difficulties in evaluating the results of reports however carefully they are designed and however well the reporter is instructed. However, some measure of agreement about the best and the worst nurses can usually be established.

Having established criteria for selection the next stage consists in finding tests or other methods of assessment which might enable the hospital to select potentially suitable candidates and reject unsuitable ones. Such tests have been developed by asking students to undergo extensive psychological investigation soon after arrival. Results of these investigations were kept and checked later against the students' progress. Several types of investigation are possible and are described below.

1. *Interviewing*

This is the most popular of all methods yet it is probably not the most effective. At an interview one person, or perhaps a committee, endeavours by questioning and assessing the answers, to gain an impression of the candidate's personality. Appearance, bearing, speech can be noticed from the candidate's behaviour. Questions can be asked about attitudes and interests and many answers allow the interviewer to gain some knowledge of the candidate's emotional approach. Interviewing can be very effective provided it is well prepared and the questions asked cover a wide area in order to make possible an assessment of all aspects of personality.

There are great drawbacks, however, in this method. Interviews take place in stressful circumstances and great skill is needed to put a candidate at ease. The interviewer's manner, facial expression, attitude of approval or disapproval may influence the candidate's answers. It is difficult to avoid asking leading questions and candidates often try to give the answer they think may be the expected one. Only a very long interview could give a comprehensive picture of the candidate's personality. In business, interviews are sometimes conducted over lunch and the more relaxed atmosphere and unbusinesslike setting make it possible to cover ground far beyond the immediate questions of work. On the whole, while some people are shrewd interviewers the method has little to recommend it. Some people believe that the interview helps the candidate more than the employer in enabling the former to see the place of work, ask questions and feel more at ease by the time work begins. Interviewing techniques can be greatly improved by training and by introducing structure into the interview.

2. *Performance Tests*

Some of the characteristics required in a nurse can be assessed by psychological tests specifically designed to do this. Accuracy, speed, perseverance, manual dexterity are some of the personality characteristics for which tests have been devised. If high scores on certain tests are obtained by students who later prove themselves to be successful, low scores by those who give up training or prove to be poor nurses, the tests are said to correlate highly with success or to have a high predictive value.

So far no tests have been found to predict satisfactorily success in nursing as distinct from success in examinations. More research is needed involving the use of 'test batteries', i.e. a large number of varied psychological tests. These will have to be used on large numbers of new recruits to nursing. Recruits must be in training long enough to make it possible to know which nurses are successful on the wards and in the school, which nurses are poor and fail to make the grade. The test battery results should then be statistically analysed.

By such methods useful tests are sometimes found which, however, may not appear to have any obvious connection with the ultimate tasks. A test consisting of holding one leg up a few inches above a chair, for example, was shown to have a high correlation with success in some jobs. It emerged that this test measures the personality characteristic of perseverance. No one could have predicted the validity of this test.

Tests of this kind probably could not be used on their own in selection because students might have little faith in them.

3. *Miniature Situations*

It is sometimes said that the only real way of knowing how suitable a person is for a job is to let her try it for a while. There are many reasons why this practice is not desirable in selecting student nurses. It is expensive, disrupts people's plans and is most distressing to those who are not successful. Instead it may be possible to devise miniature situations which resemble the real tasks a nurse may have to carry out. Her manual skill, speed, ingenuity might be tested by asking her to move or clear away some equipment. Her ability to work with others can be tested by giving a group of candidates a group project to carry out. This may reveal who assumes leadership, with how much authority they state their views, how easily they co-operate with others or how submissive they are.

Emotionality can be tested by giving conflicting instructions, criticising performance, stressing the importance of failure. Some tests of this kind have been successfully used in the selection of officers in the Services. Too little is known about personality requirements in nursing to be able to use such methods without much more research.

4. *Questionnaires*

This is by far the most common tool in personality measurement. Questionnaires are quick to apply. A great deal of information is rapidly available. The subject simply reads through the questions and puts the appropriate mark against each. Some questions require the answer 'yes' or 'no' and space is left for the expression of doubt. There are question-naires in which the subject is required to underline statements with which he agrees, cross out those with which he disagrees, leaving blank those about which he feels doubt or indifference. Answers to questionnaires can be readily checked and scored objectively, rendering interpretation by the tester superfluous.

SOME EXAMPLES OF THE TYPE OF QUESTIONS USED IN PERSONALITY INVENTORIES OR QUESTIONNAIRES

1. Are you inclined to keep quiet when out in a social group?   Yes   No
2. Are you more interested in athletics than in intel-lectual things?   Yes   No
3. Do you adapt yourself easily to new conditions?   Yes   No
4. Do you have frequent ups and downs in mood?   Yes   No
5. Do you usually take the initiative in making new friends?   Yes   No
6. Would you rate yourself as a lively person?   Yes   No
7. Do you prefer to work alone rather than with people?   Yes   No

EXAMPLES OF SELF-RATING TYPE OF QUESTIONNAIRE

In your own opinion, which of the following words apply to you? Underline them and use two lines for emphasis. Put a cross, or two crosses, through any that do not apply. Leave the rest blank.

hardworking; businesslike; energetic; steady; lively; impulsive; easygoing; unobservant; aimless; untidy; ambitious; pushful; determined; serious; self-reliant; quiet; shy; hesitant; sensitive; moody; discontented; cheerful; self-confident; popular; a leader; tactful; critical; rebellious; solitary; worrying; humorous.

Many people feel that reliance cannot easily be placed on the answers given in self-rating. The desire of the subject to put himself in the best possible light always influences the answers. More serious still is the fact that the same question may lead to very different interpretations. Some personality inventories, for example, ask, 'Do you feel diffident when you meet strangers?' As it is impossible to know how diffident other people feel and as everybody feels diffident at times, any one person may quite honestly say 'yes', though he only rarely feels diffident; or answer 'no' because he does not always feel diffident. If questions are carefully worded and well selected, however, questionnaires can have a very high degree of validity. In fact it is not really necessary to examine the meaning of the answer at all. The value in questionnaires lies in comparing the answers many people give to the same questions. Some personality characteristics such as neuroticism, introversion and extraversion can be assessed with considerable success by the use of questionnaires.

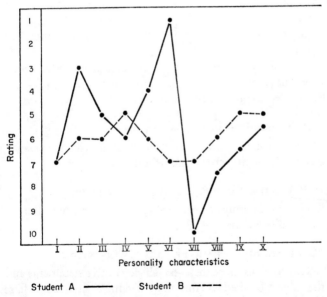

Student A ———   Student B ———

Fig. 5. Example of personality profile.

From the answers people give to questions in personality inventories it is possible to draw a 'personality profile'. This shows to what extent various personality characteristics are present. Each characteristic could be plotted on a 10-point scale, for example, and a person's profile might look something like the one shown in Fig. 5. Some personality inventories have been so extensively used that norms for the general population are now known and also the characteristic profiles for various subgroups within the general population. Profiles of nurses can then be compared with those of other people. In order to use personality inventories in selection procedures it is necessary not only to compare personality profiles of nurses with other occupational groups, but also of successful and unsuccessful nurses, profiles of young nurses and older ones, of student nurses, staff nurses and ward sisters and of nurses who have specialised in some field of nursing, for example in psychiatric nursing, theatre nursing or intensive care work.

The following are some of the personality inventories which have been used in research in nursing but so far this has not led to any conclusive results:

THE EYSENCK PERSONALITY INVENTORY

This is a short questionnaire and measures two personality scales only—extraversion and neuroticism.

R. B. CATTELL'S 16 P.F. TEST (Personality Factors)

This test measures 16 personality factors, including dominance and emotional stability.

MINNESOTA MULTIPHASIC PERSONALITY INVENTORY

This contains more than 400 self-descriptive statements and the subject is asked whether these statements are true or false if applied to himself. The scales on this test measure adjustment to family and to people of other races, and emotional stability as compared with groups of mentally ill people.

5. Projective Tests

These tests make use of people's tendencies and willingness to make up stories about things they see. When shown an ink blot, for example, people see butterflies, dancing girls, pictures of skeletons or many other images. When a vague picture is shown depicting, for example, two people a story can be invented about their relationship to each other, their difficulties and troubles. The stories people make up about pictures reveal something about their own personality; they project onto the picture feelings and thoughts of their own. The projective tests most commonly used are the *Rorschach Test* and the *Thematic Apperception Test*. Projective tests will be referred to in the chapter on perception. In nursing suitable pictures might be devised to test attitudes to patients, work or hospital.

In summary this chapter has shown how a psychological knowledge about personality measurement could help in achieving better selection of nurses. In the first instance it might be possible to find among the applicants those who are likely to be successful and to reject those who seem very unlikely to succeed. As more knowledge is gained it might be possible to discover those whose special aptitude is for special fields of nursing, such as public health nursing or psychiatric nursing.

So far the techniques of personality assessment have been applied only to the selection of nurses in a few hospitals and in an incomplete manner. Full investigation of personality is a long and expensive procedure and, perhaps for this reason, not widely practised. In other fields of work much more extensive studies have been carried out.

The two stages of fitting people to jobs and of finding

suitable jobs for people involve the use of various techniques for the measurement of personality. The first stage consists in applying tests to existing nurses and finding measurements to determine what kind of personality is possessed by the best and the worst nurses. The second stage consists in applying suitable selection tests to candidates.

There are many more uses for the personality studies described in this chapter. Reporting or interviewing, for example, enters into many situations between nurse and patient. Much of the information sought from patients is obtained by the use of questionnaires. Research into the effect of some drugs may necessitate the use of attitude tests. Projective tests are frequently used in the investigation of psychiatric illness. Rehabilitation of disabled patients may be facilitated by the use of good aptitude tests.

An understanding of the essentials of personality testing as applied to her own selection for nursing should enable the nurse to apply this knowledge where it concerns other people.

SUGGESTIONS FOR FURTHER READING

ALLPORT, G. W. *Personality*. London: Constable, 1938.

CATTELL, R. B. *The Scientific Analysis of Personality*. Harmondsworth: Penguin, 1965.

EYSENCK, H. J. *The Structure of Human Personality*. 3rd ed. London: Methuen, 1970.

HALL, C. S. and LINDZEY, G. *Theories of Personality*. New York: Wiley, 1970.

LAZARUS, R. S. and OPTON, E. Jr. (Ed.). *Personality*. Harmondsworth: Penguin, 1967.

SEMEONOFF, B. (Ed.). *Personality Assessment*. Harmondsworth: Penguin, 1970.

VERNON, P. E. *Personality Assessment*. London: Methuen, 1964.

19. LEARNING

Throughout training the student nurse learns new skills, new facts, new attitudes. Some of the learning takes place without effort by doing the job; some of it is the result of her tutors' teaching, some the result of her own study. It is helpful to know something of the psychology of learning in order to make the best use of the available time.

Learning is the acquisition of a new and better adapted pattern of response. Changes in circumstances make old behaviour ill adapted and new responses must be learnt. The home method of making beds or preparing meals is ill adapted to hospital use—new methods must be acquired. Old emotional responses to sickness are not helpful to the patient, a new approach to sick people is learnt. Old beliefs about illness prevent proper observation. New knowledge of physiology, psychology, pathology makes good observation and nursing possible. We can only say that learning has taken place if the new patterns of behaviour are an improvement on the old. If, after a period of practice, we make more mistakes than before we would not consider that learning had occurred.

Knowledge of Results

It is essential to *know the result* of learning: first, to know what kind of behaviour it is aimed to achieve; secondly to know during learning what progress is being achieved.

Many experiments in learning have been carried out on animals. Rats have been observed learning a path through a maze or pressing levers in a cage. Cats have learnt to get out of puzzle boxes, monkeys have learnt to use tools. In each case the animal knows of his success because he is rewarded with food at the end of his trial. Human learning does not always lead to such clear-cut results. Learning how to nurse leads to the patient's comfort, to better observation of the patient's symptoms, to skilful handling of equipment, but it is not self-evident from the task itself when learning is completed. Outside information must be given; for example, the patient must say that he feels more comfortable, or his evident relaxation shows it, or the ward sister's approval indicates it. Opportunities for learning are so great in a hospital that learning is almost inevitable. However, opportunities of acquiring wrong methods or attitudes are as numerous as opportunities of learning the right thing. To a very large extent what determines success or failure is knowledge of results. No opportunity of informing students of their progress should be lost. This needs to be done personally. Published results of examinations are of doubtful value especially to the less successful student. Knowledge of results fulfils two functions: it allows the establishment of a measure of learning, in other words a criterion by which the outcome can be judged, and it serves as a reward. Because of our need for approval we feel rewarded when someone praises our efforts.

In simple learning experiments it is possible to study the effect of reward on the rate of learning. A stop-watch can be used to show how long a rat takes for each successive run through the maze. The reduction in time is a measure of learning, the final stage is reached when the rat is able to run through the maze without losing its way and in the shortest possible time. The rat can be rewarded with food when he takes the right turn, punished with electric shocks at the wrong one. The effect of reward and punishment can be seen in the progress the rat makes. In human beings praise is one of the few possible rewards; very few people other than small children will accept food or sweets as reward. Praise, approval, knowledge of results act at the same time as an incentive to learning and a measure of the success achieved.

There are some situations in which progress can be measured directly. When poetry is learnt, for example, it is clear that learning has taken place when the poem can be recited without a mistake. Mistakes are easily discovered so that knowledge of results is inherent in the learning process. In learning to play tennis some mistakes are self-evident and improvement occurs as these mistakes are corrected. Failure to hit the ball or to return it into the court are obvious mistakes. Other mistakes, however, cannot be noticed by the player himself; they must be corrected by an observer: posture, the method of holding the racket, footwork, shoulder movements improve only as a result of comment from a coach.

Most learning in nursing is rather like this. Only a few mistakes are glaringly obvious and can be corrected by the student herself. Improvement in approach to the patient, accuracy in reporting, gentleness in handling, are only possible if someone draws attention to these matters. Left to herself the student may believe she is doing well. When her errors are corrected and made known to her there is a temporary setback affecting speed and overall efficiency; the next stage is a higher level of performance. Knowledge of results and awareness of mistakes are so important in learning that they cannot be overemphasised; yet, strange as it may seem, some nurses are reluctant to criticise and many other people forget to praise the work of others. Of the two, praise is probably the more important and effective.

Learning consists in making a new response to a stimulus to which it was not originally made. Rats, for example, know how to press a lever even before the learning experiment. They are learning if they manage to press the lever in response to a new situation. One experiment may consist in learning to press the lever when shown a circle, but omitting to do so in response to a square. Human beings know how to walk or speak or lift up a bowl. The nurse has learnt something new when she walks to the patient in response to a groan that previously she would not have noticed; or when she says the right words to comfort the patient or to inform the doctor; or when she hands the doctor an instrument in response to a sign from the ward sister—a sign that previously she might not have understood.

There are basically three ways of learning to match new stimuli to old responses:

1. Conditioning.
2. Trial and error learning.
3. Learning by insight.

Conditioning

Conditioning was first described by the Russian psychologist, Pavlov. He experimented on dogs. Dogs, like other animals, salivate when they eat or smell food. Pavlov rang a bell when food was offered to the dog and before long he was able to show that it was possible to produce salivation by ringing a bell without giving any food at all. After a period of ringing the bell without offering food the newly acquired pattern of salivation again stops. To maintain it it is necessary to give food again at the sound of a bell from time to time. We say that the conditioned response has to be *reinforced*. It is possible to reverse the learning process by *deconditioning;* for example, by giving an electric shock with the ringing of a bell. The association will then be with pain rather than food.

Watson, a psychologist of the behaviourist school, showed that it is possible to condition children in the same way as dogs. He conditioned his own child to become afraid of furry animals by frightening him with a loud noise every time he played with a previously beloved furry toy.

Pavlov and the behaviourist psychologists have studied in detail how conditioning depends on the time interval between the unconditioned response and the new stimulus and how conditioning is affected by reinforcement. Only a few conditioning experiments with human beings can be carried out in laboratories. It is possible to condition a blinking reflex to stimuli other than movement near the eye and it can be shown that people differ in their responsiveness to conditioning. This represents one of the differences in personality. In everyday life it is probable that quite a lot of conditioning takes place. Some psychiatric symptoms may be the result of conditioning. Fear of open or confined spaces, of sharp objects, of blood, of carrying out certain treatments may have occurred as a result of conditioning without a person's knowledge.

Aldous Huxley describes in *Brave New World* how, in his phantasy, children could be conditioned against the use of books. His method is well described though not foolproof. It is possible that some isolated, strong dislikes or phobias have accidentally occurred by this process. A systematic attempt to decondition by making new associations with pleasurable stimuli may help to overcome the symptoms. Patients have been helped by this method to overcome disabling fears of open spaces or of sharp objects. Enuresis can be relieved. Some success has also been recorded in the treatment of alcoholism and of sexual deviation by the reverse process, of establishing a conditioned link between nausea and drinking or sexually deviant behaviour.

Trial and Error Learning

Trial and error learning is best demonstrated by animal experiments. A cat which is shut in a cage can be observed to move about the cage apparently aimlessly. It touches and presses various parts of the cage; repeats, without any apparent pattern, some of the positions and actions already tried out; and eventually, apparently accidentally, hits on the right method of unfastening the door and getting out of the cage. The total time taken and the number of errors can be measured. If the cat is returned to the cage and the whole performance is repeated a slightly shorter time is taken to find the way out. Eventually the correct move is made immediately.

In the course of learning wrong moves far exceed correct moves in number as they occur many times in each trial, while the correct move is made only once at each attempt. This shows that the frequency of carrying out an action is less important than the success of it. The wrong actions serve the purpose of encouraging further attempts. Adult human learning rarely appears to take place as aimlessly as trial and error learning in animals. When we try to solve wire puzzles we come nearest to apparently aimless fiddling with the pieces until they suddenly come apart. In this manner children learn to take things apart and to fit them together again.

Learning by Insight

When the period of aimless activity is reduced to a minimum we speak of *learning by insight*. Adults, who try to take a piece of machinery apart, look at it for a long time, note pattern, screws, holes, wires and eventually, when they begin to work, they make the correct move at once and move the appropriate parts. They understand the task and know in advance which action is likely to lead to success. Even if a mistake is made it is not corrected by aimless activity but by renewed reflection until a new idea occurs.

Köhler has demonstrated learning by insight in monkeys. The monkey in the cage was surrounded by boxes and sticks of various sizes. Bananas were placed somewhere just out of reach of the monkey. By the use of boxes and sticks they could be fetched down. The monkey learnt to climb on a box to get the bananas from the roof, or to reach for them with a stick when they were outside the cage. There was often a period of unsuccessful reaching for bananas followed by a phase of apparently aimless play with boxes and sticks. Then quite suddenly the monkey piled up the boxes in the correct manner and fetched the bananas. One monkey, who had apparently given up his attempts to get bananas, played with two sticks and apparently accidentally fitted them together to make a long stick. He immediately jumped up and tried to get the bananas. He had *insight* into the relationship between the newly learnt skill of fitting sticks together and his previous attempt to obtain the bananas. Learning by insight is much more important to human beings than trial and error learning.

When general principles are used to solve specific problems insight is necessary. In working out the area of a square, oblong or triangle, the general principle is learnt and applied to the different shapes. Those children who fail to understand attempt each new problem as if it were unconnected with anything that they have learnt before. Geometry to them becomes a great burden. Measurement of dosages of drugs, or dilutions of lotion are approached by some nurses in a trial and error manner causing great anxiety in the process. Insight into the problem means that the correct solution can be found in a flash. In applying knowledge of physiology to the understanding of diseases or knowledge of a familiar procedure to attempting a new one insight learning takes place. It is possible that insight learning is similar to trial and error learning except that errors are eliminated by thought rather than by action. Instead of actually walking through every blind alley in a maze we can look at a map and think about walking through the maze. We can find the correct path before entering the maze. Similarly, we can see the correct solution of a puzzle by trying all other solutions in imagination. We can start spring cleaning in an orderly, planned way, having eliminated superfluous moves by thinking about them.

There is, however, a difference in the mechanism of various forms of learning. Some learning involves the formation of some kind of link or connection between different ideas or actions. The order of movement in bedmaking needs to be established and followed precisely so that on every occasion the same sequence of movement is carried out. Connections between words and their equivalents in a foreign language must be learnt by forming appropriate links; multiplication tables are another example. In this kind of learning 'associations' must be formed.

Some people try to learn most things in the same manner, by deliberately forming associations between one bit of knowledge and the next. They try to find ways of memorising by using mnemonics, rhymes, jokes, or they sometimes try to remember the initial letters. This type of learning is rather like learning by conditioning: new stimuli are connected with the responses to an old one. Experiments in trial and error learning or in 'rote' learning help to point to some rules of how associations are formed. Broadly speaking 'frequency' and 'recency' of association help. An association which has occurred recently is better remembered than an earlier one. The most important factors, however, are success and meaningfulness and these are associated with insight.

Insight learning occurs suddenly. It consists in seeing how the various elements of the situation are related to each other. There is a mental reconstruction until it suddenly fits. Problem solving is an instantaneous activity. For a long time the student cannot see the solution, then suddenly it is perfectly clear. Everybody has undergone this experience but it is difficult to analyse because it is so sudden.

It might be argued that a problem does not really exist until the solution is at hand. If a small child finds himself among a lot of tools and electrical equipment he has no problem because he does not know at all what the material is for. If he gets a chance he plays separately with the wires, the screws and the tools, but he does not appreciate their real function. An electrician confronted with the same amount of equipment has a problem. He sees the connection between the items and sees how electric wiring can be fixed up. He mentally rearranges the heap of material until he suddenly sees the correct way of producing a meaningful pattern.

It is clear that in nursing the student becomes aware of more problems as she gains knowledge. Each problem exists only for those who make an attempt to solve it. For the junior nurse there are no problems of ward administration. She is concerned with her own work and her problem consists in arranging her own actions or the equipment she herself uses in order to arrive at a satisfactory outcome. The ward sister sees the work of the ward as a whole. Her problem is related to her awareness of the work of all nurses and the needs of all patients.

The matron's problems refer to the interrelations between departments. She sees, organises and reorganises in her thoughts the demands of administrative, medical and domestic staff. She sees the work of the various departments in relation to each other. She takes into account total man-power, money, time. What is a problem to her is no problem at all to the junior student because she cannot see what is involved. It is not that the matron's problems are more difficult to solve than those confronting students but rather that these are problems for the matron because she is already beginning to see their solution whereas the student has not even become aware of such complexities.

Political and social problems come into existence only when we already begin to see our way to solve them. While poverty is considered to be a necessary and inevitable state of affairs it presents no social problem. When we see that it can be alleviated we become aware of it as a social problem. To small children or unintelligent people racial issues, armament, refugees, religious intolerance present no problems. They are only seen as problems by those engaged in finding a solution.

The *Gestalt* school of psychology is particularly interested in the way in which insightful learning and problem solving depend on the spontaneous awareness of the relationships of things. The German word *Gestalt* means 'form' or 'configuration'. Gestalt psychologists point out that awareness of form is an immediate experience. Perception of the total form occurs instantaneously, for example we perceive the figure of a square instantaneously, we do not build it up from 4 lines, 4 right angles. We arrange things into patterns and groups until they fit into a scheme we can understand. Learning consists in reconstructing the field until a configuration of the right sort is perceived. Gestalt psychologists stress that our behaviour is always determined by the way in which we see and understand things rather than by the objective reality of the situation. Our interpretation of environment depends on our attitude, our aim, our previous learning. We make the present fit in with our own frame of reference and the situation becomes meaningful according to our own previous knowledge.

Gestalt psychologists describe this in a vocabulary borrowed from physics. They say that we move in a 'field' according to the forces which operate at a given time. Our action may be the 'resultant of a number of vectors' leading in different directions. Barriers, whether real or imaginary, cause change in the direction of activity. They may be so strong that they counteract movement or they may result in detours or in changes of aim.

Conflict situations are described in the same graphic way: they are represented by vectors acting in opposite directions. There may be 'double approach', a conflict situation in which two alternatives appear equally desirable. This is easily solved if one force is slightly stronger than the other or if conscious deliberation gives one alternative a little more force. The choice between attendance at a cinema or theatre is an example:

$$\text{Theatre} \longleftarrow \text{Subject} \longrightarrow \text{Cinema}$$

Desire to go to the cinema moves the subject towards it. Desire to go to the theatre moves him in the opposite direction. He will soon find a way of increasing one or the other force and making a decision.

Double avoidance is a state in which both alternative actions are equally distasteful:

$$\text{B (dentist)} \underset{\longrightarrow}{} \text{Subject} \underset{\longleftarrow}{} \text{(toothache) A}$$

The individual feels pushed towards one alternative, A; but the nearer he gets to it the more he is repelled by it and pushed towards B which also repels with intensified force as it is approached. The toothache, A, pushes the individual towards the dentist, B, but the approach to the dentist makes him prefer the toothache and pushes him back again. Distaste for war may be as strong as fear of being a coward. The thought of fighting makes a man want to run away; the idea of running away is so repulsive that he feels compelled to stay.

'Approach–avoidance' conflicts imply ambivalent feelings to the same situation. Desire for an apple from the larder and fear of punishment represent such a conflict. The wish to qualify as a nurse and to pass examinations may be counter-

acted by the fear that the examinations may be too difficult
and failure may be humiliating.

$$\text{Subject} \xrightarrow{\hspace{2cm}} \text{Apple}$$
$$\xleftarrow{\hspace{2cm}} \text{Punishment}$$

Graphic representation of the conflicts helps a person to
understand that there may be complete inactivity if the forces
acting on him are equally matched. Vacillation may occur or
some people completely avoid the conflict by indulging in
totally irrelevant action. People with hysterical illness solve
their double avoidance conflict by 'forgetting'. A patient who
suffers from amnesia cannot remember who he is, what he
is doing, where he is going: he has 'left the field'.

When insight occurs learning is sudden and apparently
effortless. Students, however, are aware of the great effort
involved in study which precedes the very rewarding experience of sudden insight.

Experiments have been carried out to investigate how
learning takes place and how study can be effective. The
difficulties of experimenting with human beings are quite
considerable. If they learn too fast one cannot observe the
learning process. If one experiments with learning material,
which is familiar to some subjects but not to others, results
cannot be compared. If, for example, one were to experiment
with the learning of poetry one might find that one person
already knows the particular poem, another, though not
familiar with this poem, knows many others and learns
poetry as a hobby, a third person knows no poetry at all and
dislikes the idea of learning it. The method of learning used
during the experiment would contribute less significantly to
success than previous experience.

It is therefore important to carry out learning experiments
with tasks which are equally unfamiliar to all subjects. The
material must lend itself to measurement and must be learnt

sufficiently slowly to make observation of progress possible. The results obtained from learning experiments apply also to other forms of learning.

Learning Skills

Learning Curves

Experiments in learning skills have yielded some useful knowledge. Skills like typewriting, tracing patterns while looking into a mirror, or fitting various parts of equipment together, have been studied. These lend themselves to experimentation because learning is obvious. It can be measured by timing the total performance. A graph can be plotted showing how much more quickly each attempt was completed than the previous one. An alternative way of measuring learning is followed when a fixed amount of time is allowed and one measures how much of the task was completed: for example, how many words were typed in a period of ten minutes. Another method is to count mistakes and observe their reduction in successive trials.

These experiments have shown that learning takes place fairly rapidly at first and that there follows a period in which apparently little progress is made; then, suddenly, rapid progress occurs again. There are characteristic learning curves: a rapid rise followed by a *plateau of learning*. Depending on the complexity of the task there may be more than one plateau (see Fig. 6). One possible explanation of the plateau is that separately performed items of the skill are in process of integration. During early learning they are performed consciously. During the plateau they become habitual and form an integrated high-order form of behaviour which later allows for a new skill to be attempted. Boredom or fatigue may be responsible for plateaux.

Learning to drive a car is a clear example of this process.

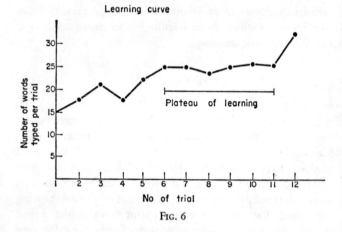

Fig. 6

Rapid progress is made in the first few lessons in the use of gears, clutch and steering. Then for many weeks there seems to be a standstill. Suddenly the whole process of using controls becomes one: gears are changed correctly without the learner being aware of it; clutch, brake, accelerator are used without conscious awareness. The driver is now free to learn the more complicated manoeuvres or to attend to traffic.

Learning to type begins with a rapid increase in the skill of using the fingers and remembering where the letters are. Then there is a plateau followed by a phase of learning in which the student is no longer aware of looking for letters but instead thinks of groups of letters and words. After a further plateau it becomes possible to think of the subject matter being typed and the typist is no longer conscious of the use of the keys.

Skills in nursing are probably learnt in the same way. The first blanket bath takes a very long time. Every action, every move is conscious. Skill in handling water, soap, flannel, rapidly increase; and after a plateau in learning the procedure is carried out sufficiently automatically to enable all the attention to be devoted to the patient without the nurse having to think which way to wring out the flannel. It is important to practise nursing procedures often enough to reach the stage at which the nurse becomes free to give full attention to the patient's comfort and need. Unfortunately, sometimes students forget that the purpose of learning a procedure is to be able to carry it out really well and they sometimes feel that as soon as they have learnt a procedure it is beneath their dignity to perform it and it becomes the task of a more junior nurse. Patients often comment on the pleasure of having a bed made skilfully, of having pillows arranged and sheets smoothed and of being skilfully lifted and placed on a bedpan. They feel this is done very differently by the ward sister and by an inexperienced student.

Plateaux in the learning of motor skills arise for other reasons also. A skill like 'giving an injection' appears to consist of a sequence of small steps in the motor performance, steps which can be practised individually and then put together into a complex task. However, the difference between the final polished performance and the early trials is not only one of speed. A number of factors apply more specifically to skill learning than to other forms of learning.

Firstly, although we refer to 'motor skills', the task is in fact a sensorimotor one. The learner must pay attention to stimuli—some from his environment, for example from the patient's facial expression or posture, some from the tools he is using, and some from within his own organism. Recognition of appropriate stimuli, and learning to exclude those which are not appropriate, takes time and some of the plateaux of learning are associated with this appreciation of redundancy in the sensory input of information.

Secondly, any complex skill consists of a number of subskills. It may be that one of the subskills is particularly difficult to perform and learning of the total skill can not progress until the subskill has been mastered. Some student nurses, for example, have particular difficulty in manipulating the clamp on a pair of artery forceps. They cannot progress with the procedure until this has been mastered.

Thirdly, the smoothness of the skilled performance arises because attention is paid to the next stimulus while the motor task related to the previous stimulus is still taking place. The skilled nurse, for example, already looks at the prescription sheet while she attaches the needle to the syringe. The learner is, at first, only able to attend to one stimulus and respond to it at that time. To anticipate the next move the way the skilled person does, practice during a plateau of learning is necessary.

Lastly, in all motor performances, minor errors occur which require correction. If one has moved the piston up a little too far one pulls back a little to correct this. Awareness of one's own performance is referred to as 'feed-back' and feed-back leads to correction. The unskilled person tends to over-correct, with the result that the performance appears jerky. Tiredness also has this effect and so do drugs and alcohol, as was shown in investigations on drivers and pilots. It seems that in spite of the fact that student nurses often find it boring, skills need to be practised in a laboratory situation before they are carried out on patients.

Everyone knows the discouragement of being on a plateau of learning. No progress seems possible, the student feels that effort is futile. He often gives up the attempt to learn if there is no one to provide the necessary encouragement to overcome it. It may well be that some of the wastage in student nurses occurs at a time of plateau. The first plateau may be reached early in the first year of training, another one usually occurs early in the second year. People often abandon their attempts to study a foreign language, or tennis, or typing, or pottery just after the first rapid progress, during the first period of standstill. Evening classes suffer a rapid reduction in numbers after Christmas, often when people feel they are making no progress and come to the conclusion that their effort is not worth while. It may be helpful at such times of discouragement to know that plateaux invariably occur and that this is not a reason for despair.

Very often a sudden increase in learning occurs just before the end of the practice period. When a learning experiment is carried out warning is sometimes given that time is nearly up: 'Only two minutes to go.' This usually results in a sudden spurt of rapid progress. Everyone is aware of the amount of learning which can be fitted into a very short space of time before examinations. There is usually some guilt feeling about doing so much in so short a time, having done so little before. This is not justified. In fact the long period of apparent inactivity is probably necessary to make rapid progress possible in the end. Some people feel that cramming before examinations is not real learning. It is real in the sense that it marks a steep rise in the learning curve, but it needs consolidation later. To avoid discouragement it is well worth while to provide periodic goals in the form of test papers or end-of-term examinations. These are valuable in terminating plateaux. Obviously they would lose in value if they occurred too frequently. The spacing of intermediate goals should depend on the age of the student and on the subject matter. (Children need them more frequently.) The degree to which morale is influenced by a feeling of despondency where no progress is made should also be taken into account.

Laws of Learning

Most learning is not learning skill but information and facts. This depends very largely on insight. To investigate learning more accurately experiments have been carried out which aim to measure the acquisition of insight, for example, experiments on concept formation. Other experiments set out to investigate laws of learning.

The most comprehensive series of investigations was carried out by Ebbinghaus. He used nonsense syllables in his experiments. These syllables are formed by picking out vowels and consonants and putting them together in such a way that they have no meaning: GEZ, LEB, SIL, KES, would be acceptable syllables; SUN, DOG, BUT, would be excluded because they have meaning. Nonsense syllables can be arranged to form lines and groups of lines to be learnt like poetry. They can be presented visually, given to the subject to read and study, or they can be projected onto a screen one at a time, or exposed in an apparatus for a measured length of time or read aloud to the subject. Ebbinghaus investigated the effectiveness of the various methods of presenting material in learning.

The first step in the experiment consisted in deciding how to measure learning. It is possible to measure how many syllables have been learnt in any given time. Another possibility is to measure the time taken until the subject is able to repeat the assignment correctly. Using this as a measure of learning it is found that, although the subject was able to repeat the material correctly immediately after learning, he quickly forgot. If asked an hour later he could remember only very little of it, the next day hardly any at all. If on the next day, however, he relearns the same material he does it much more quickly than the first time, showing that learning had not been completely wasted.

Measurement of forgetting and time saved in relearning is as useful as the observation of learning and mistakes. Even if the subject remembers none of the material he learnt the previous day he may be able to pick out of a number of sheets of paper the one he had studied the day before; he recognises what he has learnt. Recognition is an indication of learning. The only way the subject could manage still to remember his assignment the next day would be to go on learning long after his first accurate reproduction. This is called *over-learning*. We do this with poetry or with parts in a play; we repeat them many times after we have first succeeded. Most other learning does not proceed to the point of over-learning because most people find it boring to go on with something they feel they know well. It follows that in order to know a subject well it must be relearnt after some forgetting has taken place, or so much more must be learnt in the first instance than is really necessary that there is still enough knowledge left after forgetting. Relearning is the usual practice in school and in nurse training. However well a student knows the subject at the time she learns it she has to relearn before each examination. She may feel disappointed when, at the end of a year, she feels that she knows less than she did at the end of the Preliminary Training School. But on relearning she finds it possible to reach her original level in a very much shorter time than before. Even the vaguely familiar ring of some things apparently completely forgotten is a sign of learning and a help in relearning.

Textbooks and lecturers usually give much more information than the student needs, allowing for a good deal of forgetting. Some students find very condensed textbooks helpful, but for most students these are useful only for revision purposes. They cannot easily be used for study because there is nothing to spare for forgetting.

Ebbinghaus tried various arrangements of nonsense syllables to see in what order people were able to memorise the material. He found that the beginning and the end were learnt most easily and also any syllables that were markedly different from the rest; for example, if any of them were presented in red, while the rest were black, these were remembered easily. If any of the syllables are accidentally meaningful, for example if one of them belonged to the learner's own car number or telephone number, these too will be learnt quickly. Learning, then, spreads from the quickly learnt parts to the parts immediately in front and behind and so on until it is complete.

Similar ways of learning are often observed in real situations. The first and last lectures of a course often stand out; so does any lecture given by a visiting lecturer or a substitute. If any lecture happens to be particularly relevant to the work the student is just doing in the ward, or to a patient she happens to be nursing, it is much better remembered.

In any one lecture the opening remarks and the summary at the end are the really important parts. Any anecdote told in the middle is also likely to be remembered because it stands out. Methods of study were investigated by Ebbinghaus. He found that if a one-hour study period was divided into six ten-minute periods with intervals much more learning took place than if the hour was undivided. He referred to this as *distributive* learning. It is more effective than *massed* learning. This applies to many other learning situations. At school, for example, four periods of mathematics per week are better than two double periods or one whole morning. The time-table for student nurses is usually so arranged that each subject is taught on every school day rather than a whole day being devoted to a single subject. Some people believe that a course of lectures spread over perhaps twelve weeks is more useful than if all lectures are given in four weeks and for that reason they find study days more effective than study blocks. Private study should be distributed over several periods in preference to a few long sessions. One hour's study every day is better than two days of staying up all night. It is more effective to study a little of each subject every day than to devote one evening to anatomy and physiology, another to public health and yet another to psychology. There is, of course, an optimal study period for each type of subject matter. Where a large amount of preparation is necessary, for example if apparatus has to be set up as in bacteriology or for physiological experiments, or in practical nursing, it becomes uneconomical to make the class too short. Lectures are better used if they are as short as possible. Each student must find his own best rhythm for study, but however convinced an individual may be that she studies best by sticking to one subject for many hours it is at least worth trying to divide the total period up into several shorter ones and to distribute them more evenly over the weeks or years.

Ebbinghaus showed that there was a marked difference in the rate of learning according to the method by which the total amount was tackled. In some instances his subjects were encouraged to learn a page of nonsense syllables by reading through the whole lot and learning the whole page. In other instances the page was divided into several parts, each part being learnt separately. The former method is called *global learning*, the latter, *part learning*. Global learning is more effective than part learning. Although many subjects believed they could succeed better if they learnt a few lines at a time they did, in fact, learn more easily when they treated the whole page as one. In learning poetry the method of learning one verse at a time leads to an association of the last line of the verse with the first line of the same verse instead of leading on to the next. The result is that the first verse is very well learnt, the rest much less so and that there is a risk of getting stuck and having to restart instead of being able to carry on when prompted. It is particularly true that a meaningful whole is more easily learnt than separate parts which do not appear to have any meaning in relation to each other. The whole poem, not its separate verses, has meaning. Even with nonsense material wholes are learnt better than parts; difficult parts need special practice later.

To apply the principle of global learning to the study of

nursing it is important to consider how big the 'whole' subject should be to make a suitable unit for learning. Lecture courses can be so arranged that the first lecture gives a survey of the total subject to be covered and the last lecture gives a summary of the course. Any individual lecture can in the first few minutes give an outline of the subject as a whole. Textbooks are sometimes so arranged that the first chapter gives an indication of the total subject matter of the book. Each chapter has an introduction giving an outline of the whole chapter. In this way each part is seen in relation to the whole. It is worth while beginning a new subject, anatomy and physiology for example, with a very simple outline of the total functioning of the body. Reading a very simple book like those written for children, which can be read through as a whole before detailed study of any part takes place, can be helpful. Most students find it difficult to learn any part of physiology when it is first attempted. After a study of the whole body the study of any one part falls into place and becomes quite easy.

One of Ebbinghaus's most important findings relates to the contrast between *active* and *passive* methods of learning. He compared the results if the subject spent all his time reading the material to be learnt with the effect of spending part of it reciting the material himself. Learning takes place much more rapidly if the subject attempts actively to recite after every reading. Many other learning experiments confirm this. If a person tries to learn vocabulary in a foreign language it takes him much longer to go on reading the words and their translations than to try to think of the foreign word then look it up if he fails. The activity of searching for the answer helps him to remember it when it is supplied.

This principle applies also to nurse training. In the course of study it is essential to do something actively about the information in the books or that derived from lectures. During a lecture, for example, it helps if the student listens actively and applies the information while it is being given. Some people write it down and feel that the activity of writing while listening makes them active. It would probably be more useful if they wrote only an occasional note because this might involve the greater activity of evaluating what is said, sorting it and selecting from it what appears worthy of a note. If the lecture refers to some patient whom the student has nursed it is useful to think actively of the application of the subject to the work she has seen in the ward. Throughout a lecture she should listen critically. This does not necessarily mean looking for faults though that can be a very useful activity. A critical approach may mean admiration of the skill with which the subject is treated, or comparison of the lecturer's methods with those of others. It involves a silent running commentary on what is said. Textbooks should be read with the same critical approach: as the student reads she can actively discuss with herself the meaning of the statement, the method of explanation and its application. Reading rapidly and actively summarising is much more helpful than reading slowly and trying to remember.

Silent discussion with oneself is one way of learning actively. More useful still—whenever it can be done—is discussion with others. Asking questions, explaining to others, giving a talk oneself, repeating to someone what the lecturer has said, are the best ways of learning. Active methods of learning may involve trying to discover an answer to a problem oneself before the answer is given by the teacher or by the book. This is why some teachers begin by asking questions even though they know that the students probably do not know the answer. If the students try to find out first they are more likely to make full use of the explanation when it is given. Writing papers is an essential tool in the clear formulation of thought. The most fruitful method of learning is an attempt to communicate to others what has been learnt. Reporting back, either by a straightforward summary or in some more dramatic manner, such as enacting some point in a sketch or putting it into poetry helps one to learn it.

Motivation for Learning

All learning depends on motivation. Only if one wants to learn can learning take place. Human beings want to learn for a variety of reasons: in childhood, because they want to please someone; later, because self-respect is enhanced by success. Knowledge may seem worth possessing for its own sake. Children show immense curiosity and explore endlessly, repeating any action which gives unexpected and pleasurable results. They will, for example, switch lights on again and again once they have accidentally discovered how switches work, continue to pull the lavatory chain, or repeat words or syllables which sound pleasing to them. Many adults find success in learning sufficient motivation. Success in nursing patients well, in doing work well in the ward, is sufficient motivation for those who want to nurse to make them persevere with the difficult and sometimes uninteresting parts of their study. Where additional motivation appears necessary it is interesting to consider the effect of reward and punishment as incentives to learning.

Rewards can be tangible: sweets or presents can be given, but adults do not often need this. For most people praise acts as a reward. Punishment can be physical, though this is hardly applicable to adults. It can consist in some enforced deprivation. For most adults, criticism and blame act as punishment.

Experiments have been carried out chiefly with animals where reward in the form of food or water is not only an incentive to learning but the end point of the learning experiment. Experiments with children are more relevant. In one of these experiments carried out by Hurlock groups of children were learning arithmetic; without actually checking on their results first one group was left to carry on without any criticism or encouragement. Children in a second group were repeatedly told how good they were; those in a third group were told how stupid and lazy and incompetent they were. The results showed that the group who were given neither reward nor punishment progressed least of all. Both the rewarded and the punished children improved at first, but very soon there was a marked falling off in the group who were criticised and a steady improvement in the group who were praised. It is generally found that punishment has only a very transient effect and only if, by improvement, there is hope of earning praise. Punishment has been found effective in 'avoidance' training, but otherwise constant punishment without rewards for effort has no beneficial effect. Encouragement and praise, on the other hand, are incentives to do well either in order to retain the good opinion of others or because of the pleasure obtained from work well done. Praise must be sincere to be effective in the long run; indiscriminate praise can be effective only in a short experiment.

Learning is made easier by working with other people. In some experiments the progress of several groups of children was compared. Some children worked by themselves, some worked in different rooms but knew that other children were working elsewhere, and some worked in direct competition with each other.

Those who competed did best, but even working in company with others, or in awareness of others, was better than working entirely alone. The usefulness of competition and rivalry is well known to students. Provided the members of the class are well matched and all have an opportunity to be successful competition is encouraging. If students are of very differing ability some are bound to be unsuccessful however hard they try and, for these students, competition is discouraging. Their incentive to learn may have to come from competing against themselves, trying to improve on their own previous performance.

Much attention has recently been paid to the use of teaching machines and to methods of programmed learning. In these systems the material is presented to the student in small amounts. Before he is allowed to proceed he must give the correct answer to a question based on the text he has just learnt. He benefits from the immediate knowledge of results and from the rewarding experience of being right. The success of this method of learning in other fields suggests that there may be some useful applications to nurse training.

SUGGESTIONS FOR FURTHER READING

BORGER, R. and SEABORNE, A. E. M. *The Psychology of Learning.* Harmondsworth: Penguin, 1966.

GAGNE, R. M. *The Conditions of Learning.* New York: Holt, Rinehart Winston, 1967.

HILL, W. F. *Learning.* London: Methuen, 1964.

KAY, H., DODD, B. and SIME, M. *Teaching Machines and Programmed Instruction.* Harmondsworth: Penguin, 1968.

LEGGE, D. *Skills.* Harmondsworth: Penguin, 1970.

MACE, C. A. *The Psychology of Study.* Revised ed. Harmondsworth: Penguin, 1968.

20. REMEMBERING, FORGETTING, PERCEIVING

Learning depends, among other factors, on two important activities:

1. The way in which new material is first apprehended, that is, the process of perception.
2. The amount of forgetting which takes place.

A small amount of information can be retained for a short period and recalled perfectly. A telephone number for example which one has just looked up is retained long enough to obtain the connection. If, however, the number is engaged one may have to look it up again before dialling a few minutes later. This process of remembering events just perceived is referred to as 'short-term memory'. The short-term memory has, however, only very small storage capacity. It has been suggested that approximately 7 items can be held in the short-term memory and recalled. If the input is greater then information is either forgotten or coded for transfer to the long-term memory. To retrieve information from there is difficult. Although storage capacity is thought to be virtually unlimited the process of 'remembering', i.e. bringing back into consciousness the relevant items of information accurately and speedily is rarely achieved with perfection.

In this chapter only long-term memory will be discussed.

Some forgetting is inevitable. It is most rapid at first and takes place more slowly as time goes on. Immediately after the first correct repetition of a poem or a series of nonsense syllables forgetting begins. One hour later only a small amount will be recalled, two hours later there will be still less recall, four hours later even less and by the next day there may be

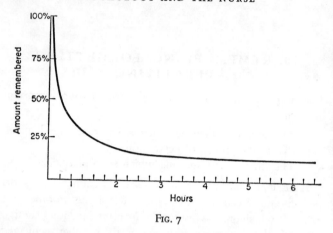

FIG. 7

very little. The difference in the first few hours is very marked. It then becomes less noticeable and barely matters after several days. The amount recalled is illustrated in Fig. 7.

The amount of forgetting can be reduced by over-learning in the first instance; that is, continuing beyond the moment of first correct recall. Many lessons at school and in nurse training aim to do this by spending more time on every subject than appears necessary to the student. Forgetting is also allowed for by going more deeply into every subject than is really essential, ensuring that, even after forgetting a good deal, enough is still remembered.

Students often guard against forgetting by thinking about the material at intervals, in fact by relearning at odd moments. Forgetting is least marked if, immediately after learning, the student goes to sleep. The next best activities following learning are games, sports and relaxing at social activities. If it is necessary to learn several subjects it is best to follow any period of learning with a subject of a completely different nature. Forgetting is most marked if two subjects learnt in succession are very similar to each other. Experiments with nonsense syllables show that the worst possible results arise from learning several groups of nonsense syllables in succession. Syllables followed by groups of numbers produce much better results; shapes or drawings make a better contrast still and relaxation or sleep after learning gives the best results of all. School time-tables are so arranged that a language lesson is followed by mathematics, not by another language; history is followed by physical training, not by geography or literature.

Variation of subjects is carefully arranged in nurse training schools so that very dissimilar subjects follow each other; for example, practical nursing and anatomy. In her own study the nurse can use her time in such a way that the greatest possible variation occurs. A period of reading may be followed by writing or discussion, the greatest possible variety of subjects being studied in succession.

Remembering depends not only on how well the material has been learnt but also on the extent to which remembering is useful. As soon as any knowledge becomes superfluous it tends to be forgotten. If the student works for examinations only and cannot see the usefulness of her knowledge in her work then most of what is learnt is forgotten immediately after the examination. Information about individual patients is remembered until it is used either for reporting or in treatment. It is forgotten as soon as use has been made of it. Remembering incomplete tasks and forgetting completed tasks results in great economy of effort and allows us to take in new information all the time, which would be impossible if every bit of information no longer needed were still retained. Student nurses can be helped to make the best use of their experience by being shown how each piece of knowledge forms part of a bigger whole and therefore continues to be of use. Anatomy and physiology for example are not subjects to be learnt and forgotten when no longer needed. They are learnt in order to make use of them later in the study of disease. Knowledge gained about one patient does not cease to be useful when the patient is discharged. It becomes useful when it is applied to the nursing of some other patient with a similar complaint or a similar personality and when lectures about the patient's disease are attended or textbooks are consulted. Lectures can be so arranged that each subject remains open for the addition of more information and thus forgetting can be reduced. It is helpful to end a lesson knowing where the information leads, or aware that information so far obtained is incomplete. A lesson which leaves the student sufficiently dissatisfied to cause her to reach for a textbook in search of knowledge, or which has aroused sufficient interest to lead to discussion, is much better remembered than a lesson which is well rounded off and complete in itself.

Forgetting is often associated with the learner's emotional state. Everybody tends to forget unpleasant, painful experiences. This process is called repression. This is not a conscious process and is a great help in dealing with unpleasant experiences and with any less desirable personality characteristics. Not only the unpleasant experiences are forgotten but also the anger, sorrow, humiliation which accompanied the experience. If learning becomes an emotionally unpleasant activity forgetting is much more pronounced. This may be why punishment is not in the long run effective in promoting learning. Experiments with incomplete tasks show the process of forgetting very clearly.

In one experiment children were given a large number of tasks to do, each taking only a few minutes. They were allowed to complete some and in others they were interrupted before they had finished; for example, there were a few lines to be copied, a few sums, some drawings to be copied, codes to be deciphered and many other tasks. At the end the children were asked if they could remember the things they had been asked to do. They remembered only some of the tasks and this depended on the instructions they had received. Those who were told in advance that there would not be time to complete them all remembered the incomplete tasks and forgot the completed ones. Some had been told that the whole thing was very easy and had been made to feel stupid for not completing the tasks. They remembered only the completed ones and forgot the unfinished ones about which they felt uncomfortable.

A similar experiment was carried out with adults who were asked to do some puzzles. Some were told they were testing the puzzles in order to grade them according to difficulty. Others were told that all the puzzles were very easy and well within the capacity of small children. The subjects were not allowed to complete some of the puzzles. Those who thought they were testing the puzzles remembered clearly the unfinished ones. The others, who felt that they were stupid because they had not succeeded in all the puzzles, forgot the unfinished ones and remembered the completed ones.

The forgetting of unpleasant, worrying events is sometimes evident when a history is taken from a patient. Some of the most significant events in the patient's life may be completely forgotten. A serious illness, a stay in hospital, or the causes of his parents' death may not be recalled by the patient. Even prompting by a relative may not lead to recall. Without knowledge about repression it would be surprising that such important events should be forgotten.

Repressed material is not necessarily permanently forgotten; it may be inaccessible to conscious recall at one time and may be remembered quite spontaneously in a different context. In fact, conscious effort to remember may make it more difficult. Free association of ideas may suddenly lead to the recall of something which appeared to be completely forgotten and which, when remembered, arouses considerable emotion. Repressed material is recalled when current events and circumstances evoke a connection and when the emotional state makes it possible to remember. When anyone is depressed or hears depressing news all past recollections suddenly assume a depressing nature. All kinds of examples of the sad things that have happened to the individual himself, to others, to the world are suddenly remembered. When the mood is good, funny or amusing incidents, jokes and success stories are remembered. It is well known that visitors to patients sometimes indulge in recollections of all the sad and unfortunate experiences which they remember suddenly when the association with hospital, sickness and death brings those memories to the fore. Patients do not find stories of other people's suffering, operations, treatments and misfortunes at all comforting. Nurses may have to help visitors to remember positive, encouraging, hopeful topics of conversation by their own cheerful, optimistic attitude to visitors. The visitors in turn help the patient to think of cheerful events in response to their mood.

Repression of unpleasant, painful thoughts occurs not only about the past but also about the future. For many patients the problems related to their return home, resuming the role of the breadwinner and the position in the family usurped by someone else during his illness, are so difficult that they rarely emerge in consciousness.

The patient may appear to forget his family and his work and remember only events which occur in the hospital. His conversation is about the ward, the nurses, other patients, the food he is served, the activities of doctors, matron and other staff. He appears to forget all he is told about his own home and family. Children in hospital show this to a very marked degree. They appear to forget their parents soon after arrival in hospital, do not talk at all about home and sometimes fail to recognise their mother when she visits. It is very obvious that the thought of home would be too painful and is therefore repressed. Rehabilitation is very difficult until the patient is able to think of his future life. It becomes possible to help patients once they consciously worry about specific problems or difficulties, but no help can be given while the patient has apparently forgotten all about his troubles. Repression of painful material is a useful defence mechanism, allowing the patient peace of mind and relaxation. It is a solution of difficulties in so far as it makes the patient behave as if these did not exist. To overcome difficulties, however, the patient has to be helped to face them. In the long run protection from the recall of unpleasant thoughts is not in the patient's interest.

The activity of remembering is only possible if the brain is healthy and intact. When the brain is damaged by accident, operation, drugs or toxins remembering is impaired. The amount of forgetting is related to the extent of the brain damage. Because forgetting takes place most rapidly immediately after learning, before consolidation has taken place and much more slowly later on, the material most recently learnt is most completely forgotten after head injury. Old knowledge remains intact. After accidents causing unconsciousness there may be complete loss of memory for the events leading up to the accident. Patients who suffer from concussion may have forgotten what they were doing at the time of the accident. On recovery from electroconvulsive therapy, epileptic fits or an anaesthetic the patient may forget where he placed his belongings, what was the last meal he ate, which part of the ward he is in.

Some forms of brain damage interfere not only with recall but also with ability to understand and learn what is going on. Old patients, or patients who suffer from confusional states during heart failure or fever, appear to suffer from loss of memory for recent events while retaining vivid and detailed memories of their distant past. Their inability to remember recent events is very largely due to their lack of attention and concentration and consequent failure to grasp and learn what is happening around them. Accuracy of remembering depends first and foremost on the accuracy of observation and on the learning which take place in the first instance.

Some people have the ability to see every detail instantaneously. They succeed in taking in a complete picture at once as if they were storing a photograph somewhere inside them. Later, when trying to remember, it is as if they were looking at the photograph and reading off details they might not consciously have noted at all. This process is called 'eidetic imagery'. It is a rare ability, useful to anyone on whose accuracy of evidence one has to depend. It occurs more commonly in children and in some artistic people. Most people perceive only inaccurately what is happening and their ability to remember reflects faults in perception in an exaggerated way.

Perception is the interpretation of sensory stimuli which reach the sense organs and brain.

The eye is capable only of distinguishing shape, movement and colour. When we say that we can see a table, or Uncle Jack, or a boat on the horizon we make use of the sensations, remember other similar sensations and give a meaningful explanation of them by referring to objects and people.

Perceiving is a learnt activity. To perceive it is necessary to remember previous experience and to recognise the new sensory stimuli as identical or similar to stimuli previously experienced and named. When the infant first experiences the sensory stimulus which an orange, for instance, presents, a coloured round image appears on the retina. Similar images are produced by the moon, a large ball or a rattle. Later the infant repeatedly has the same sensation but he learns to handle the orange and gets an idea of its size. He puts it into his mouth and learns about its texture, he smells it, bites it and learns about taste, throws it and learns what weight it has and how much damage it can do. Eventually, he hears the word orange frequently used in connection with the object and learns that it can be cut and produce a good drink and that his mother does not like him to play with it. When he then *perceives* an orange all his knowledge about oranges is used to interpret the visual impression.

The moon, which at first produced the same stimuli, has not given any new information. It cannot be reached or played with, knowledge about it remains much more imperfect than knowledge about oranges. Perception of distance, however, has been learnt by the fact that the moon cannot be reached.

The ball and the rattle are recognised by the noise they make, the texture when they are pressed or sucked, their hardness. Their size is known by handling them; and their distance, when they are first seen, is realised by the effort required to reach them. Playing with them is approved of and encouraged. By the time the infant can name the four different objects which produce the same orange, round, visual image he is making use of a wealth of information without being conscious of it. Perception includes all this information.

All perception is learnt in the sense that we can name what we perceive only if similar perceptions have occurred before. The use of language is closely linked to perception.

From an assortment of separate perceptual events we begin to extract characteristics they have in common and then use a symbol, for example a word, to refer to the objects with which we associate these common properties. Such symbols are called 'concepts'. Concepts are not static. Once we begin to use a concept our perceptions are organised in new ways. The concept helps us to 'generalise', i.e. to try to apply the concept to new and different perceptual patterns, and then to 'discriminate', i.e. to eliminate inappropriate objects from the class embraced by the concept, by becoming aware of specific perceptual patterns on which to base the classification.

When something entirely new appears we can only describe it as being '*like something else*', possibly like a composite picture of a number of previously known things. We can perceive the new thing only by comparing it with what is already known. At the moment of perception an effort is made to make the experience meaningful. This 'effort after meaning', as it is called by some psychologists, determines the way in which the experience is later remembered. If, on first acquaintance, a man looks like 'Uncle Jack' he is remembered to be like him. When asked for details later the colour of his hair is given as dark, like Uncle Jack's, he is remembered as having a moustache like him, as about six feet tall, of medium build. His eyes, mouth, smile, movements are recalled as resembling those of Uncle Jack. In fact the more the new acquaintance is thought about the more like Uncle Jack he appears to be. Often when the new acquaintance is seen again one fails to recognise him because in reality he may be very little like Uncle Jack while the memory of him has become more and more similar to Uncle Jack.

Perception depends always on one's degree of understanding at the time. As everybody who perceives the same thing has different previous knowledge, different expectation and attitudes, different standards of comparison, no two people ever perceive the same event in precisely the same way. In remembering what was perceived distortions occur according to the importance that has been attached to the various parts of the perception in the first instance. In some ways it is remembered as being more conventional than it really was; in other respects unusual details, which had been noticed, are exaggerated on recall. Different people's reproductions of the same situation in paint or drawing or in story form are totally different.

The psychologist, Sir Frederick Bartlett, has demonstrated the process of perception and the distortion in remembering by a series of experiments. He drew a pattern, for example, which had certain features of a cat but otherwise was a very unusual design. The first person to be shown the picture was asked to draw it from memory and pass his drawing on to the next person who, in turn, drew it from memory. The features resembling a cat became more and more cat-like until in some series a completely conventional drawing of a cat was produced, often with cat-like details totally unwarranted by the original picture. Other reproductions stressed some of the unusual features of the design and these were accentuated until there was a cat with patterns specifically noted to be unrelated to the cat. Both the familiar features and the unusual ones had become exaggerated.

Similar distortions occurred in the retelling of a rather involved, illogical story. Familiar elements were retold in more and more familiar versions. The story became shorter, more logical and more commonplace. A few details seen to be incongruous became more absurd and irrelevant.

It is very important to remember the distortions which occur in perception and in subsequent remembering when the reliability of evidence is considered. What is seen at the time depends on what the observer expects to see, on his attention and on the meaningfulness of what is perceived. How much of it is remembered, and how accurately, depends on the distortions which take place in the effort to understand. It also depends on a person's emotional need to forget unpleasant aspects, particularly as they affect him himself. It is very easy for him to accept suggestions as to what he has perceived and then to believe it to be his own perception. After being shown a picture for a short period the subject can be asked to describe what he has seen. When he has enumerated all he can remember, some of which is almost certainly wrong, he can be asked such questions as: 'Did the lady in the picture wear a hat?' or 'How many bottles did the milkman carry?' Even if there was no lady or milkman in the picture many people are prepared to give the number of bottles and to swear that the lady did wear a hat. They later remember the lady and the milkman perfectly clearly. If they are shown the picture again they are genuinely surprised to find how different it is from their recollection. It is well known that distortion occurs when people give evidence in court. Counsel for defence or prosecution make use of this knowledge when they wish to throw doubt on the reliability of evidence of a witness.

Nurses have to learn to perceive some situations accurately and guard against distortion in reporting. Signs and symptoms of the patient, his facial expression, posture, abnormal colour, or observation of pulse, of excretions or discharges cannot be accurately perceived by the new student because she does not know what to expect when she looks at the patient. When she knows something of the illness she notices symptoms which she has learnt to look for. Her observations become meaningful. The more experienced and knowledgeable she is the more detailed the perceptions become. Because observations become more meaningful they are better remembered and reported. Unusual or unforeseen events, such as accidents or sudden changes in the patient, are less well perceived because the necessary 'set' to make perception meaningful is lacking. It is all the more important for the nurse to give a running commentary to herself at the time, making details of observation conscious and writing a statement immediately, before distortions can occur. One can train oneself to observe by noticing what belongs together, what is out of place, what changes are taking place and what explanation of them might be given.

Training nurses to perceive details and remember accurately depends on knowing what is relevant. The new student cannot distinguish, among a mass of details, those which are relevant to the patient's illness. The more experienced nurse uses a 'concept' and therefore selects perceptions relevant to the patient's illness. There are obvious advantages in being able to select what is important, but also dangers, because knowing what to look for makes it possible to neglect observations which appear irrelevant yet may be significant. This is why a fresh look at the patient, the unbiased report of a new nurse, the observation of another doctor, the comments of visitors may bring to light some symptoms which had been overlooked. Sometimes the fact that the patient's illness has been 'diagnosed' interferes with observation. Only those things which are relevant to the named illness are noticed, other symptoms or complaints may be ignored and a better understanding of the patient's illness prevented. Transfer of the patient to another ward, or the introduction of new staff, may lead to a completely new way of looking at him. The publication of articles describing a new syndrome often leads to many observations of the condition, because attention has been drawn to symptoms previously thought to be irrelevant. An attitude of optimism and hopefulness leads to observing improvement which might go unnoticed in a more pessimistic setting.

Although perceiving is a learnt activity there are certain stimuli to which we appear to respond more readily than to others. Some noises cannot be ignored, some patterns of sound are noticed with more pleasure than others. Some visual stimuli tend to call for response more readily than others. Gibson, for example, has shown that even small infants respond to depth cues and keep away from a cliff.

McDougall included in his definition of instincts the tendency to pay attention to stimuli of a certain kind. Animals respond in a specific way to some selected stimuli. Birdsong, coloration of the male animal, certain movements of the body for example, evoke sexual behaviour. Some objects, for example feathers, grit and straw, are perceived by birds and used for nest building. Birds respond to particular patterns on the mother's beak and peck at it. Certain specific patterns of stimuli are perceived as a whole and act as 'Innate Release Mechanisms' (a term coined by K. Lorenz) for the animal's instinctive behaviour. It is difficult to find similar specific patterns of stimuli in human beings. However, there is apparently a tendency to perceive some kinds of pattern with satisfaction while other stimuli appear to us to be defective and unsatisfactory.

We notice things which have a good form and have a tendency to distort perception in accordance with our expectation of good form. Squares, circles, symmetry are perceived with satisfaction. Figures which are well rounded and closed are more pleasing than irregular shapes with parts missing. 'Gestalt' psychologists pay particular attention to the need for completeness, wholeness and closure. Our need to see figures as if they were complete leads us to ignore faults at times. We see this shape ⌐⌐ as a square and remember it as a square without paying attention to the missing lines. When we do notice that a piece is missing the gap is magnified in our perception and recollection because it is disturbing to feel that the figure is incomplete. When nurses observe symptoms they tend to observe all the symptoms which should be there, although some may be missing.

When observations do not fit into a good pattern we have a tendency to make up a pattern. We remember numbers in groups, make up rhymes, make noises into tunes. Similarly we try to classify observations. The greatest satisfaction is gained when everything is neatly organised and named. Our tendency to organise perception into a clear pattern is so great that we sometimes feel satisfied when order is established, without realising that the organisation into pattern stems from us not from the material we perceive. We feel satisfied when we know the name of a disease without realising that the disease for which we have only one name may in fact have many causes, many different origins, many manifestations, that, in fact, there may be many conditions grouped together under one name. Nurses often believe that they know more about the patient when they know the diagnosis. In fact they have merely satisfied their need to categorise. In order to know more about the patient it may be necessary to forget the classification and look again at all the details which can be observed.

The need to classify, to see things as complete, to close the subject, is much greater in some people than in others. The activity of creating order from a wealth of apparently unrelated perceptions is a valuable step in acquiring scientific understanding. However, to see clear patterns where they do not really exist, to demand simple structure always, and to see things only in clear categories, leads to an excessively simplified perception of a complex situation; it prevents reassessment and regrouping of perceptions and means that a great deal of material is ignored. Learning consists both in the activity of creating clear, classified patterns which serve as a framework for further perception and learning, and also in the process of reconstructing existing patterns, reassessing and breaking down established patterns to make integration into bigger wholes possible.

People who are particularly keen to establish clear and simple structures are said to be intolerant of ambiguity. Adorno and Frankel-Brunswick have shown that in extreme cases such people are apt to impose their simplified classification system also on moral and social issues, that they tend to be prejudiced and are said to have an 'authoritarian personality'.

To a lesser extent, however, all people are engaged in attempts to reach clear structuring of their perceptual world and to defend the understanding of their concepts from the disruptive effect of new perceptions which do not fit in. Festinger studied what he termed 'cognitive dissonance', a kind of disharmony one experiences when new information makes it difficult to persevere in one's attitudes and beliefs. When such information is supplied in the form of new perceptual cues, these tend to be either distorted or ignored.

The ability to reassess and reclassify material diminishes in old age and is sometimes impaired when a person has suffered head injuries.

When we perceive the world around us we always have to make some judgments on rather scanty evidence. Often we do not even know why we judged as we did. Size and distance of objects, for example, are related to each other. We know how big people are. When we see them as being very small we judge them to be a long way off; when they look big we think they must be close by. We use a 'frame of reference' of well-known objects and judge new impressions by comparison. We assume, for example, that the walls and window frames of a room are vertical and judge people's position in space by reference to the room. If the room is distorted we tend to misjudge the size, distance and shape of objects and people in it. When we know the shape of an object, for example when we know that the table top is square, we continue to see it as square whatever the position of the eye, and therefore the image on the retina, may be in relation to the object. We tend to see colour as constant even if the light changes.

There is always the possibility of error in perception. We usually compensate for errors by using several senses at the same time. We do not rely entirely on sight to judge size and distance, but also use touch and hearing. We verify the perceptual experience by handling the object and doing something with it. Very often, however, errors in perception do occur; these are called 'illusions'. Some of them are universally experienced, some are personal errors resulting from private expectations and attitudes. Some visual illusions can easily be demonstrated and examples may be seen on page 276. Perception of size is often determined by the importance attached to the person or object. Children nearly always see and remember their teacher as being tall and big. An experiment with similarly sized coins of different value showed that the coins of bigger value were seen to be bigger than the coins of smaller value. Villages, towns, places known in childhood appear bigger in retrospect than they really are. Holidays appear longer than they really were.

Sometimes it is difficult to know how much error there is in perception particularly if there is no means of checking by a different approach. In familiar surroundings it may be easy to recognise shapes or noises. If the frame of reference is removed it may be impossible to perceive accurately what is going on.

Many patients find it very difficult to distinguish clearly what they see and hear in hospital. Where everything is strange and new there are no fixed impressions against which to measure the reality of perceived events. This is made worse by any defect in vision or hearing the patient may have. It is a terrifying experience to be unable to orientate oneself clearly. It cannot be stressed too much how important it is to help a patient to learn about his environment by making use of every possible sensory device. Showing, allowing the patient to touch, to handle and to use equipment, explaining,

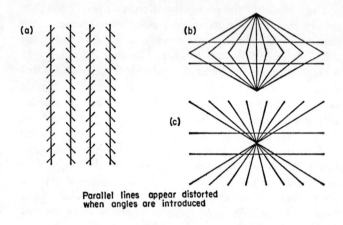

Parallel lines appear distorted
when angles are introduced

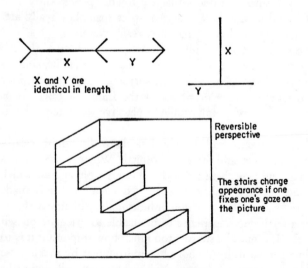

X and Y are
identical in length

Reversible
perspective

The stairs change
appearance if one
fixes one's gaze on
the picture

FIG. 8. Some examples of illusions.

talking about the tools used to carry out a procedure, confirming the patient's perceptions when he is right, correcting them when he is mistaken, are essential to good nursing. Particular attention must be given to a patient whose eyes are bandaged, who cannot hear clearly, who is only partially aware of his environment because of sedation or whose position in bed makes it difficult for him to observe what is going on.

Perception is the necessary raw material of thought. If a person is deprived of sensory stimuli it becomes very difficult for him to think clearly. Images of previous perceptions become so important that it is hard to know for certain what is reality and how much comes from one's own reconstruction of past perceptions. Normally we can clearly distinguish between images and reality because images belong to one sense only. In the absence of sensory stimulation images become so powerful that they begin to be taken as perceptions.

There are some mentally ill patients whose own images are so powerful, even when they perceive reality, that they fail to distinguish between reality and images. The term 'hallucination' is used for perceptual experiences which do not arise from sensory stimulation. It is never possible to be sure whether a patient is misinterpreting a stimulus and has an illusion, or whether he experiences a perception for which there is no stimulus at all—a hallucination. Some patients are able to describe their hallucinations very clearly, either in words or by drawing pictures of them.

We often manage to have fairly accurate perceptions even though the stimulus is very weak or present for only a very short time. We refer to the perceptual threshold when we try to measure how long an exposure is necessary before a picture or word is recognised, how bright the light has to be before we can see, how loud a noise must be to be heard. The threshold differs for different people. Activity of the sense organs plays a part. Apart from that the individual general state of readiness and awareness determines the threshold of perception. When a person is tired or ill the threshold may be high and many things he would normally notice remain unseen or unheard. Certain drugs, however, heighten perception. Aldous Huxley described the changes in perception which occurred when he had taken the drug mescaline. Some people, who have become addicted to drugs, have perhaps done so because they enjoyed the greater awareness of stimuli under their influence. The threshold for hearing may be lower when other senses are not used. Blind people can learn to make use of auditory information which is not noticed at all by sighted people. It is possible that patients in a stupor have a much lower auditory threshold than is realised.

The threshold differs for familiar and unfamiliar stimuli. Those stimuli which cause emotional distress differ from those which are neutral. Nurses sometimes become unaware of noises which are clearly perceived by and are very irritating to patients. The sounds of a trolley being set up, of keys rattling, may be very alarming to the patient and not observed at all by the staff. Conversation between nurses or between doctors is often heard by the patient to whom it refers, just as anyone may hear his own name mentioned against the general background of noise of undifferentiated talk. Patients always believe that preparation for treatment or discussion of prognosis or diagnosis refers to themselves and, therefore, hear and see clearly some things which in isolation give rise to misunderstanding and unnecessary anxiety.

Although conscious perception occurs only when sensory stimulation has reached the threshold of perception a certain amount of information can be conveyed by noises or visual stimulation just below the threshold of the individual. This is referred to as 'subliminal perception'. It can be demonstrated that words of a given length, printed sufficiently clearly and largely, can be read when they are flashed momentarily on a screen. At that point words which have no particular emotional significance can be clearly recognised. If words which cause anxiety—referring to death, violence, suffering or sex—are interspersed with neutral words it is found that they cannot be recognised at that level of exposure. The threshold of perception for these words is higher than for neutral words. Measurements of blood pressure, breathing, perspiration, however, show emotional response. This indicates that some perception must have taken place below the threshold. This can also be demonstrated if a person is asked to say the first thing that comes to his mind every time something is flashed on the screen. Even if he is not quite able to read the word on the screen the association which comes to mind is usually relevant.

The fact that some perception occurs even below the threshold of conscious awareness has been used in advertising in some countries. If the name of some merchandise is flashed on the cinema or television screen so fast and so feebly that it is not consciously recognised it is not possible to resist such advertising deliberately and therefore it may be more effective than a more overt use of advertising. Most people consider that 'subliminal' advertising is immoral. The publication of results of subliminal advertising has caused a good deal of indignation. For practical purposes it is useful to remember that whispered words, or a very brief glance at a chart or a textbook, may leave patients with incompletely understood awareness, which may nevertheless cause changes in their behaviour and emotional state.

The way in which people perceive the world around them is clearly dependent on themselves as much as on the sensory stimulation provided. Previous experiences, readiness to listen, attention, interest, physical health may make a lecture or demonstration perfectly clear to one student while another student, whose background, attention and interest differ, may come away from the same lecture with a totally different impression of what has been said. Much of what is perceived

FIG. 9. An inkblot similar to those used in the Rorschach Test.

in any given situation is in fact put into it by the perceiver. The external world is reconstructed and interpreted to fit in with the personality of the person who perceives. He is 'projecting' into the situation much of his own personality. Clearly, the more precise the external stimuli the less room for projection; the more vague the external circumstances the more projection can take place.

Projective tests can be used to give some indication of the personal element which enters into perception. Two of the most widely used tests are the Rorschach Test and the Thematic Apperception Test mentioned on page 231. Tests similar to the Thematic Apperception Test could be devised to discover a nurse's attitudes to the various situations she is likely to meet.

The way she approaches hopelessly ill patients, her reaction to death or to permanent disablement, to old people, also her way of looking at the structure of hospital administration, staff relationships, the way in which she sees her own position in the community could be elicited by use of projective tests. Projective tests cannot be very easily scored or standardised. The stories told by the subject must be interpreted by the psychologist who, in the process of interpretation, projects some of his own personality into the way he understands the stories. However, a much clearer picture of each student's individual understanding could be gained if her characteristic way of perceiving her work and her own personality could be known.

SUGGESTIONS FOR FURTHER READING

BARTLETT, Sir F. C. *Remembering*. Cambridge University Press, 1967

HUNTER, I. M. L. *Memory*. Revised ed. Harmondsworth: Penguin, 1964.

VERNON, M. D. *Psychology of Perception*. Harmondsworth: Penguin, 1965.

21. THE WORK OF SOME
WELL-KNOWN PSYCHOLOGISTS

In previous chapters frequent reference has been made to psychological experimentation. This has led to an understanding and knowledge of the laws of learning, remembering, perception and behaviour.

Only a brief summary of the main schools of psychology can be given in this chapter. Details of the experiments would go beyond the scope of this book, but they make interesting reading and students are urged to read more about them in any standard textbook of experimental psychology.

Wundt. The main influence in the early days of experimental psychology came from Germany where the psychologist Wundt began to study the measurement of psychological reaction in his laboratory. The general trend of measuring and then expressing psychological laws in mathematical form originated from this work.

Ebbinghaus and Titchener. Some of the early work on learning was carried out in Germany by Ebbinghaus and in England by Titchener. Their main contribution was the detailed description of the association of ideas. They expressed their findings in the form of laws of learning. Their method of approach is often referred to as the 'associationist school' of psychology.

Thorndike arrived at similar conclusions from observing 'trial and error' learning in cats.

Pavlov. His experiments in the conditioning of dogs and his interest in the physiological basis of behaviour led to the foundation of the 'physiological school' of psychology, a school of very great importance. It has contributed to the understanding of body-mind relationship, in other words, the psychosomatic approach to behaviour. It is possible to produce conditioned responses in human beings. Some psychologists attempt to treat certain symptoms by conditioning. Patients have been conditioned to vomit when they taste alcohol. In this way it may be possible to cure alcohol addiction.

The great school of '*behaviourist psychology*' is to some extent a development arising from the conditioning or 'reflex' school of psychology. Like the conditioning school behaviourists are interested in the relationship between *stimulus* and *response*. They are, however, more concerned with *behaviour* and to a less extent with the underlying physiological processes. Behaviourists study only *observable behaviour*. They do not deny the existence of experience, but because experience cannot be verified by objective observers or by experimentation they limit the subject matter of scientific psychology. They define behaviour in fairly wide terms Not only the gross movement of the body but also the small amount of muscle contraction, which is observable only with the aid of instruments, is taken as behaviour, so are changes in glandular function, perspiration, diameter of capillaries, blood pressure, pulse and respiration rate. These are referred to as 'molecular behaviour', while the total response of the organism is called 'molar behaviour'.

John B. Watson is considered to be the founder of the behaviourist school of psychology. He is said to have used his own child for some of his experiments and to have claimed that it should be possible to produce any desired form of behaviour by means of conditioning. In his book, *Behaviourism*, he explains the main principles of the behaviourist method of study. Most of the behaviourists have confined their experiments to animals. Some of their findings are applicable to human beings; the laws of learning, for example, appear to be very similar in animals and men.

Karl S. Lashley has contributed valuable information about the function of the brain cortex in learning. He has shown that earlier beliefs about localisation of brain function were over-simplified. He removed part of the cerebral cortex from rats after they had learnt to run through a maze. The animals had forgotten the maze after the operation but were able to re-learn to a varying degree. Their handicap in learning depended more on the amount of cortical tissue removed than on the site of the lesion inflicted on them.

B. F. Skinner has studied learning in animals in extensive experimentation. He became interested in the difference between 'respondent' and 'operant' behaviour. Respondent behaviour occurs when an external stimulus is presented; operant behaviour results from food deprivation or other internal drives. Skinner used puzzle boxes in which the animal pressed a lever to obtain its reward and procured its own food when it behaved correctly. Skinner refers to this as *instrumental* learning. The animal is instrumental in producing the effect.

Skinner has shown that learning takes place more rapidly if reward is obtained only intermittently rather than on every occasion. His methods of developing instrumental learning are applied in programmed instruction, particularly in linear programmes. The material is presented in such simple steps that the student is induced to give the correct response on each occasion and is rewarded by finding out that he is right when he reads the next part of the text. Recently Skinner's principles have also been applied to the management of mentally disturbed patients and delinquent children, manage-ment commonly referred to as 'behaviour modification'. Skinner's fictional accounts of his own theory, *Walden Two* and *Beyond Freedom and Dignity*, can be highly recommended to students who wish to think more deeply about the moral issues involved in behaviour modification.

The Gestalt School of Psychology in contrast to behaviourism is almost entirely concerned with 'experience', particularly the experience of perception which, in their opinion, is immediate and primary. For many centuries arguments had been going on about the nature of perceptions; for example how do we know that what we see corresponds to the real thing? What is the relationship between the characteristics of the external world and our sense data or between sense data and perception? Gestalt psychologists offer one solution; treating as real and important *only perceptions*, ignoring what lies behind them because it cannot be known. We behave according to our perceptions. Gestalt psychologists are also interested in the neurological events which accompany perceptions. Although there is no precise knowledge of this they believe that there is a physiological event of comparable pattern to the perception, a 'trace' in the brain. This theory is referred to as 'isomorphism'. The aspects of perception considered important by the Gestalt school are those which create patterns, order and meaning of the sensory impressions. We always experience things in a 'perceptual field'. This means that everything we see is seen against a background. The background helps to determine the figure we see.

The same object is seen as a square or diamond according to its background; or, in the language of Gestalt psychologists, according to our perceptual field (Fig. 10).

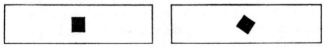

Fig. 10. An object seen differently according to its background or perceptual field.

If patterns do not exist we tend to create them: we group objects, perceive notes in the form of rhythm or a tune. The entire pattern is seen as a complete whole and can be transposed onto a different background or into a different size, or, in the case of music, into a different key. We feel more comfortable if a figure is a good one. Gestalt psychologists speak of 'good form' if it is complete, closed, rounded, symmetrical, full. Another word they use is 'pregnant' for a well-rounded, complete figure. The most important psychologists of the Gestalt school are *Wertheimer*, *Kohler* and *Koffka*.

Kurt Lewin developed the idea of 'field dynamics', transposing the idea of forces acting in a field according to definite laws from physics to psychology. The field in which we operate is our own psychological field as we see it. Behaviour can be understood if it is known how people perceive the barriers and tensions in their own life. Lewin's method of representation is helpful for our understanding of the private world of the paranoid patient. He shows how the perception of danger depends on the individual's own field and how it affects behaviour. Failure or success depends entirely on the individual's own levels of aspiration, his own field of action with its own barriers, limits and tensions rather than on objective difficulties. Other psychologists of the Gestalt school are working on problems of human conflict. In Canada the work of *Hebb* is throwing light on the physiological process of learning. Experiments with machines which can learn have some bearing on Hebb's very complex theory.

H. J. Eysenck. In this country Eysenck is systematically subjecting psychological research to statistical analysis and attempting to put much experimental work on a sound, scientific base and testing the theories of others by scientific method.

SUGGESTIONS FOR FURTHER READING

BELOFF, J. *Psychological Sciences*. London: Crosby, Lockwood Staples, 1973.

EYSENCK, H. *Uses and Abuses of Psychology*. Harmondsworth: Penguin, 1953.

EYSENCK, H. *Sense and Nonsense in Psychology*. Harmondsworth: Penguin, 1957.

HALL, C. S. and LINDZEY, G. *Theories of Personality*. New York: Wiley, 1970.

HOLLAND, J. G. and SKINNER, B. F. *An Analysis of Behaviour*. New York: McGraw-Hill, 1961.

PART III

Psychology and the Hospital

PART II

Psychology and the Disabled

22. INTRODUCTION

In previous chapters I tried to describe how a knowledge of personality development and of personality characteristics helps nurses to understand patients and themselves. Throughout these chapters, however, it was assumed that behaviour could be explained if there was sufficient knowledge available about the individual's uniquely characteristic personality.

This assumption is not entirely justified. Behaviour is not only determined by the individual's own personality but also by the standards and expectations of the society in which he lives. There is as much variation between people of different cultures as there is between different people in the same society. Whether a patient complains noisily or suffers in silence is only partly determined by his own personality. Partly he follows the standards of behaviour of his own group. In some countries people who cannot control their emotions and who give way to tears are thought childish. Those who hide their feelings are admired. In other countries it is not only proper to display feelings but if the patient does not complain his suffering may not be understood or indeed noticed.

People of different cultural backgrounds have different feelings about privacy. To some people it may be perfectly natural to undress in public, to submit to nursing care in an open ward, to be examined in the presence of a group of students. Other people value privacy and modesty to such an extent that they become acutely distressed in many situations which occur in hospital. To be seen naked even by one nurse may cause them great anxiety and physical examination by a doctor of the opposite sex or before onlookers may be quite unbearable.

In some societies it is customary for the whole family to visit the patient frequently, to crowd around the sickbed and either to try to interest the patient in family affairs or to try to share his sufferings with him. In other societies it is more usual to expect that the patient needs peace and quiet. Visitors try not to burden him with their affairs and they do not expect him to include them in his private world of suffering.

People differ greatly in their eating habits. Each nation has its own favourite foods, its own way of preparing and cooking food and its own rules about the number of meals eaten per day. It is necessary only to remember what a cup of tea means to the English to realise that some attitudes are shared by people of similar cultural background in little things as well as in big issues.

Not only national and racial culture, but also social class, determine behaviour. The middle classes, from which many nurses are recruited, share a liking for order and cleanliness which may be strange to some patients. There are differences in moral values between members of different social classes. The middle class, for example, may feel more disapproving of premature sexual relationships than either the upper or the lower classes. Attitudes to divorce or to illegitimate babies may vary between members of different social classes.

Student nurses may find it profitable to read some of the very interesting books on sociology and social anthropology. These describe widely divergent patterns of culture. The behaviour of many patients, and the attitude of some of their colleagues, may be more understandable in the light of such reading. In the next few chapters attention will be focused on the influence of the hospital culture on the behaviour of patients and personnel.

Social psychology is the study of the individual in relation to his society. It is well known that the same person may behave very differently when he is at home, at work, at his club, or a patient in hospital. The social setting and the presence of other people determine which kind of behaviour is appropriate.

Social psychologists have studied behaviour in many different situations. Few studies have been carried out in hospitals. Much more is known about schools, universities, factories and small social groups, such as family or club. An attempt will be made to examine the kind of psychological problems which are studied by social psychologists. The question of whether the findings are applicable to the special problems of the hospital will be left open until more research can answer it.

SUGGESTIONS FOR FURTHER READING

ROSE, A. M. (Ed.). *Human Behaviour and Social Process*. London: Routledge & Kegan Paul (Paperback), 1971.

WORSLEY, P. (Ed.). *Problems of Modern Society*. (Part 8, Sickness and Health), Harmondsworth: Penguin, 1972.

23. STEREOTYPES, ROLE, STATUS

People often say that they would recognise a nurse anywhere. There is a belief that membership of the nursing profession causes the individual concerned to behave differently from other people. In some instances there is truth in the statement that nurses behave in a special way; in other respects it is probably a fallacy. When reference is made to *role-determined* behaviour it is implied that certain jobs or certain positions in life are associated with predetermined behaviour patterns. When, on the other hand, there is a generalised discussion about people, ascribing characteristics to the entire group as if everyone belonging to it were alike, one is using a *stereotype* which rarely has any valid justification.

Stereotypes are over-simplifications and generalisations about national, racial or religious groups as well as social and professional groups. Many people believe that all Germans are alike, or that there are typical Chinese or Arabs or Jews. People of the upper class, or of the working class, are described in stereotypes. Nursing or teaching are professions about which stereotypes exist. When the stereotype consists of many unfavourable characteristics it is often associated with prejudice. People build an idea for themselves of the typical Jew or the typical Negro and then behave to all Jews and Negroes not according to their real personality but according to their own idea. Often people are surprised when they find that the people they meet are quite different from their preconceived idea. They tend then to call their new acquaintance atypical but to keep their idea of the stereotype intact rather than modify it in the light of experience. When the stereotype formed about a group contains fewer unfavourable characteristics it may give rise to humorous descriptions and characterisations or to unjustified admiration. There are many jokes about the British army officer, the city financier or the foreign diplomat. Some of the more eccentric aspects as well as some of the more likeable personality characteristics enter into these stereotypes. When the Germans are described as thorough, reliable, hardworking, or the Japanese as good businessmen, the Americans as efficient and forceful, the French as amorous and emotional, national stereotypes are being used.

The danger of forming judgments about whole groups of people on the basis of stereotypes lies in the difficulty this creates in communication and understanding. It is much more difficult to get to know an individual really well if he is approached with a ready-formed opinion. Anyone who dislikes all Jews and has a stereotype of Jews as mean, grasping or dishonest people is unlikely to be friendly, sympathetic and sincerely interested when he makes the acquaintance of a Jew. His relationship with the Jewish person is likely to become strained as a result of his own first approach and he will consequently reinforce his unfavourable opinion and his stereotype idea of the Jews.

Doctors and nurses have been accused of treating all patients as if they were unintelligent and socially inferior; a stereotype surviving perhaps from the era of poor-law legislation.

Stereotypes about nursing are very commonly formed in the popular mind. They do not give rise to prejudice but they hinder clear thinking and communication about nursing. The greatest difficulty arises from the indefinite nature of the concept of 'nurse' which enters into the stereotype. For most people it embodies the person who actively cares for the helpless sick, soothes the feverish brow, fights for the life of a sick child or watches over the delirious mutterings of a wounded soldier. It is not at all clear in this picture of the nurse what precise knowledge or skill she requires for her activities, or indeed what are the activities involved in fighting for someone's life. The detailed professional requirements are not included in the stereotype. Nor are the many activities of the nursing administrator, the nurse in public health, the nurse in many specialised fields of work. The stereotype of the nurse includes only the bedside nurse; not her skills, but only her personality. She is a person who is good, kind, patient, wise, alert, selfless, devoted—in some way a superior being. Sometimes the stereotype of the nurse is an exaggeration of all the positive and favourable personality characteristics people would like to find in their nurse. Often, however, some of the less likeable characteristics are added. Nurses are seen to be hyper-efficient, cold, hard-hearted, disciplinarian, authoritarian people. It seems possible to combine the most contradictory characteristics in the stereotype of the nurse.

Patients often enter hospital with a stereotype of a nurse in mind. Their idealised picture of the nurse helps them to gain confidence at a time when they most need to trust the hospital. On the other hand they may fear the nurse and react with unreasonable apprehension to the hospital. Nurses have the difficult task of breaking down the patient's stereotype and showing him that they are real people.

Nurses, themselves, have stereotypes in mind when they decide to enter the profession, which act as a model for the new student. There are a number of possible dangers. The model may be so unreal and idealistic that there is no hope of ever achieving any resemblance to it. If the student retains the idealised stereotype of the nurse, she will think of herself as a failure and become discouraged in her work. It is also possible for her to think of herself as prematurely approaching the stereotyped image. Some nurses as soon as they put on a uniform have phantasies in which they imagine themselves to be the perfect nurse they have in mind. They believe that they really are always kind, patient, helpful and knowledgeable. Such a view interferes with the examination and critical assessment of one's own personality, which is a necessary part of professional growth.

It has been found that some people are much more inclined than others to stereotype people. Those who are given to stereotyping often find it difficult to change their opinions. They have been described as rigid or inflexible in many of their attitudes.

Some interesting studies, for example those carried out by Frenkel-Brunswick and Adorno, have shown that a number of personality characteristics tend to occur together. People who form stereotypes do so particularly in relation to national, religious and racial groups and are often highly prejudiced. They tend to think well of their own social and cultural group and have a low opinion of others. They are inclined to be impatient with people whose opinions differ from theirs, they adopt highly moralistic attitudes and feel punitive to those who do not conform to their values. Such people are often found to have been submitted to hard, threatening parental discipline and approve of it. They are used to a rigid hierarchy in their family relationships and feel comfortable in a well-structured, highly organised environment. Any form of ambiguity may cause them considerable anxiety. They classify events, people and behaviour into good and bad, white and black, right or wrong and have difficulty in appreciating the wide range of intermediate behaviour. Sometimes such people are described as having an authoritarian personality.

To have a stereotype of a nurse in mind sometimes makes it difficult to understand the tremendous differences between the requirements in various branches of nursing. The hospital nurse may more or less fit the stereotype; the health visitor almost certainly does not fit it. Nurses in mental hospital work or in mental deficiency do not resemble the stereotype at all. The question—what is *real* nursing?—reveals the difficulties which arise from having a stereotype of one particular kind. It may be very difficult for a nurse to adapt herself to a new experience in nursing if she has not learnt to modify her stereotype.

Role-Determined Behaviour

A nurse's behaviour is strongly determined by the way she sees her *role* and the way other people in the team understand it. Every job carries with it certain expectations of the person who fills it. Appropriate behaviour and attitudes are prescribed. In some fields of work there are clear, written rules about the kind of behaviour which is obligatory and the kind of behaviour which is prohibited. In the army it is impossible to be in doubt about the appropriate behaviour for every occasion and for every rank. For nurses the rules are unwritten, not always clearly laid down, somewhat flexible. It is sometimes difficult even for nurses to discover what behaviour is expected of them and a great deal of anxiety arises because of the fact that an unwritten code of role behaviour has to be learnt.

When the psychologist speaks of role he does not mean to define what part of the total work should be done by any particular individual; nurses sometimes refer to roles in that sense. They speak, for example, of the nurse's role in relation to the team, meaning to define precisely which jobs should be carried out by the nurse, which by the doctor, the social worker, the occupational therapist. Or they speak of the role of the nurse in health education, trying to define for themselves what special contribution the nurse can make. Psychologists are not concerned with the definition of the scope of the work. When they speak of 'role' they wish to determine what kind of behaviour has to go with the job which has been decided upon.

With each role there are some patterns of behaviour which are essential. Others, however, appear less directly related to the work yet they are equally carefully regulated. It is, for example, essential to nursing that the nurse should be willing to preserve life, that she should have an interest in the weak, the sick, the helpless. It seems essential that she should obey orders in an emergency, that she should be willing to work at week-ends or nights at least sometimes, that she does not go off duty in the middle of an operation. All these ways of behaving are inherently related to the nature of the work.

It is much less clear why a nurse should never go off duty early even when she is not busy, why she should never smoke in uniform, why she should completely accept irregular duty hours, or why she should wear uniform at all. There may be very good reasons for each of these things, but they are less clearly related to the requirements of the work itself and constitute permitted, not obligatory, behaviour.

Other workers do not always agree with nurses about the nature of role-determined behaviour. They may, for example, find it difficult to understand the rules about smoking, or the way in which nurses defer to each other in discussions. On the other hand they may expect the nurse to perform tasks she is unable or unwilling to perform, or may take upon themselves tasks which the nurse sees as related to her role. The doctor may require the nurse to carry messages for him or to remind him of his engagements. The nurse may not see that this is related to her task. She may feel that she should give more help to the doctor during an operation; he may not see this as part of her function. The fact that no role is entirely defined leaves room for each to create his image of his own and other people's roles. There is often considerable mis-understanding and friction until open discussion clarifies the issue. While for each person the stereotype of the 'nurse' differs, the role most commonly associated with all who have the title 'nurse' is 'bedside care'; within the nursing profession, however, different categories of nurses are perceived to have different roles. Student nurses, staff nurses, ward sisters have different behaviour prescribed for them; nurses outside the ward team behave differently again. Patients are often vaguely aware of these complications. They may become very anxious if they call a nurse 'sister' or the sister 'nurse'. They are afraid to ask the wrong person for a glass of water or a bedpan and they worry because they do not know whom to ask for information. Nurses, themselves, may know that their role does not prohibit giving bedpans or whatever attention the patient needs, but the patient may not understand this. The patient may need help to understand the issues clearly and to reassure him about the fact that his care is the business of every nurse whatever her role.

To become a 'patient' also involves the assumption of a role. Studies have shown that nurses expect patients to be dependent, submissive, non-inquisitive. Patients who are seen as too independent are not popular. Neither are patients who do not get better fast enough to satisfy that part of their prescribed role.

There are occasions when the nurse's role relationship with a patient becomes an important aspect of treatment. The nurse may, for example, take on the role of mother substitute to a child or a psychiatrically ill patient. There are times when a helpless patient may regard the nurse as a mother figure, even if he is no longer young enough to need mothering. Some patients cast the nurse in the role of friend, confidante or counsellor.

The nurse's behaviour is not only determined by her role relationship with patients but also by her role in relation to other members of the staff. Within the nursing hierarchy those senior to her expect from her submissive, conforming behaviour, those junior to her expect from her the kind of behaviour from which they can gain confidence and support.

Nurses and doctors sometimes find it difficult to select appropriate behaviour towards each other. As a woman the nurse may expect from a male doctor consideration which is incompatible with his role as a doctor or with her role as a student, as a helper or as a junior member of the nursing staff. On some occasions the role expectation people have of each other is the traditional one determined by sex, age and membership of a democratic society, on other occasions role-related behaviour in hospital cuts right across normal conventions. The nurse's many roles frequently demand variations in behaviour which result in conflict and anxiety.

Status

When the difference in behaviour expected of nurses of various ranks is examined reference is made not only to role expectation but also to *status*. Status is the position of importance each occupies in relation to other people. In every group an order of importance and esteem inevitably develops. Colleagues give each nurse a certain status at work. At home in the family she occupies a different status position. People have status in their club, in the classroom or in the community. Status may be high in one social group and low in another. A father may have a high status in the family; at work he may occupy a position of low status. A child may consider his family position one low in status, but his performance at school may give him a high one there. He may have a higher status on the playing field than in the classroom. It is important to most people to feel that their status is high at least somewhere in their life. Most people are happier at work if they are satisfied with their status there.

To understand how status affects nurses' behaviour it is

necessary to examine the status of nursing in relation to other jobs and to examine the status associated with various positions in nursing. The status of nursing as a profession is frequently discussed. Many nurses feel strongly that their status is not high enough. Yet at the time of choosing their career they must have regarded it favourably. No one is likely to choose a career which he believes has low status. Some opinion surveys of the status of nursing have been carried out. Nurses themselves have been asked what occupation they would have chosen in preference to nursing and which occupation would have been their next best choice had they been prevented from nursing. This kind of inquiry reveals where the nurses see their profession in the status ladder. Some compare nursing with other professional work such as medicine or teaching. Others compare it with such jobs as secretarial or salesman's work. Men look upon it differently from women. The status which schoolteachers give to nursing determines to some extent which of the children are encouraged to think of nursing as a career.

Some people feel that monetary reward determines the status of work, or at least reflects its status. Others feel that money is unimportant in determining it, that the intrinsic value of the work is the essential factor. On the basis of the argument that the intrinsic value of work is important people responsible for the administration of the health services seek to raise the self-esteem of every group of workers by stressing their special contribution to the welfare of patients. This does not, however, entirely prevent the attempt of each group to raise its own status.

Status affects the patterns of communication which take place between people. Not only is the choice of topic restricted between people of unequal status, but there are also unwritten rules about who is permitted to start the conversation, who is responsible for bringing it to an end. Status determines the distance people keep from each other during their communication, what posture they adopt and the way they establish eye contact. When a conversation is in progress a person of higher status assumes he is entitled to interrupt; a person of lower status does not. Sometimes the fact that a person is permitted to interrupt can be interpreted as an indication of the status with which he is endowed.

Status problems within any one group may become all the more important if the profession as a whole is uncertain of its position. In nursing much of the traditional behaviour of juniors towards seniors, and seniors towards juniors, is related to status difficulties. People are uncertain whether they can retain their status in a more informal atmosphere. The whole system of hospital etiquette is designed to strengthen and clarify the status system and to make it more dependent on the job each individual holds and less on personal characteristics.

Some people find a sudden change in status very uncomfortable and distressing. Having held a responsible job before entering nursing new students may have difficulties in adjusting to student status. Each move between wards may necessitate adjustment to a new status. Work in a new special field of nursing may make the nurse feel insecure and doubtful of her status.

If patients experience change in status this may determine their attitude to sickness. Theoretically the patient enjoys the highest status of all the people in hospital. In practice patients may feel very lost because of the sudden loss of status at work, in the family and in their social setting. In hospital the patient may feel that he is unimportant. His attempts to seek attention, or his behaviour towards other patients, may represent his attempt to regain a more satisfying position. Loss of status is a particularly troublesome problem in the care of long-stay patients, especially if they also suffer from the stigma of mental illness. Goffman has drawn attention to the institutionalising effect on every aspect of the patient's behaviour if the staff assume high status positions towards him and if the patient's low status is emphasised by subtly discrediting encounters with staff. When people feel comfortable and satisfied with their status, and when they clearly understand their own and other people's roles, *morale* at work tends to be high. Morale will be discussed in the next chapter.

SUGGESTIONS FOR FURTHER READING

ARGYLE, H. *The Psychology of Interpersonal Behaviour*. Harmondsworth: Penguin, 1971.

BROWN, R. W. *Social Psychology*. New York: Free Press, 1965.

GOFFMAN, E. *Asylums*. Harmondsworth: Penguin, 1968.

KRECH, D., CRUTCHFIELD, R. S. and BALLACHY, E. L. *Individual in Society*. New York: McGraw-Hill, 1962.

NEWCOMBE, T. M. *Social Psychology*. 2nd ed. revised. London, New York: Dryden Press, 1966.

24. MORALE

When people are observed at work it can readily be seen that an atmosphere exists between people which affects their happiness, the quality of their work, their attitude to the place of employment, their work satisfaction, indeed every aspect of their working life. The word *morale* is often used for this all-pervading aspect of human relationship. When morale is high everything at work goes well. When morale is low there are many indications of disturbance. Morale cannot be directly described or measured. Instead, many different aspects of work are used separately as indices of morale.

Although there is no way of demonstrating morale its influence is felt by all members of the group. Each person is aware that his or her own attitude and behaviour are part of the characteristics of the group as a whole. Each is aware that some factors outside his own personality are affecting him. Morale is influenced by the extent to which people in the group are able to solve their problems of status and role definition. These are only a small part, however, of the total picture.

General Job Satisfaction

Job satisfaction makes for good morale and is greater when morale is high. It occurs when the work meets the needs of the people who perform it. It is not always easy to identify the needs of all the people who work together; and usually, although all have chosen the same job, they have done so for very different reasons.

People enter nursing with all kinds of preconceived ideas about the work. Often their idea of the real nature of the work has little correspondence with reality. There may have been no opportunity to find out in detail what kind of work nurses perform, what skills or knowledge are required, how much study is needed, how much money is earned; working conditions may not have been investigated and possibilities for promotion or for specialisation may never have been discussed. The nursing stereotype may be all that has guided the choice of a career. The new recruit may have matched this stereotype against her own idea about herself. Her daydreams about her own future may also have lacked factual basis for action. When the work is thus chosen without adequate knowledge about her own ability or the nature of the work job satisfaction is unlikely to occur.

Only some of the motives for choosing nursing may be consciously expressed. Some women hope to satisfy their need to give freely of their maternal feelings. Some need to have recognition and esteem, some need scope for their creative abilities and their thirst for knowledge; some seek companionship and friendship from their fellow workers; some need to feel big and powerful and hope to be able to achieve this as a result of their mastery over sickness and adversity. The need to gain independence from home may be very important. Often these needs are unconscious but may nevertheless enter into the choice of a career. Nursing can satisfy many of these needs and this is why so many people derive tremendous satisfaction from their work. Not all needs, however, can be met all the time. When some unconscious needs remain unfulfilled one tends to feel frustrated. In order to plan one's career realistically and gain maximum satisfaction from work it is necessary to become aware of unconscious motivation.

If the future nurse needs to be protective and motherly, for example, she may be happier nursing severely sick people and should not choose to work in a convalescent or rehabilitation ward. If she needs to feel challenged she might choose a situation in which frequent emergencies arise rather than work with chronically ill patients. Some fields of nursing make more demands on the intellectual ability of the nurse, others on her emotional adjustment. Success in each case satisfies different needs. Promotion to administrative posts often means reduced contact with patients and therefore less opportunity to satisfy some of the emotional needs but more opportunity to satisfy achievement needs.

There are so many different aspects of nursing that it should be possible for everyone to find satisfaction. The new student may have to be helped to see how different her experiences are in each of her successive ward assignments. While she is unaware of her own motivation she may find it hard to see beyond the current experience and if her needs are not satisfied she may feel she wants to give up nursing. Job satisfaction depends not only on the fulfilment of emotional needs but also on the extent to which the work measures up to expectations. The term 'level of aspiration' is used when one asks what aims people set for themselves.

Most people have a fairly realistic idea of their own abilities. They seek work which is difficult enough to provide continued stimulation and yet is not so difficult that it cannot be accomplished. As each person experiences success or failure he adjusts his level of aspiration. Some people's personality is such that their level of aspiration is unrealistic. Their anxiety may be so great that they always set their level of aspiration much too high, or they may have learnt, by setting it much too low, never to risk failure. People like this find it difficult to be happy and content in their work. But people who are able to set their level of aspiration realistically may also be disappointed in nursing. Some feel that there is insufficient scope for them. Circumstances may prevent them from aiming high enough or from progressing fast enough. People in senior positions sometimes discourage what they consider to be too rapid progress.

In order to work to full capacity it is necessary to have the opportunity to experiment with new ideas. One must try new skills and risk making mistakes. In nursing mistakes may, however, prove dangerous to patients and so elaborate safeguards may limit the progress the student is able to make. Most nurses enjoy the challenge of emergency situations although they may be worried by the amount of responsibility they may have to take when they feel inadequately prepared. On the whole a nurse finds it is a more satisfying experience to perform a task which stretches her ability to its limit than to work comfortably within her previous competence. Some nurses, either because they are more timid or less able, fail to gain job satisfaction because they dare not set their levels of aspiration high enough or because, however low they are set, the reward of success never comes.

When students enter nursing their level of aspiration is usually in the range of responsibilities concerned with bedside nursing. In order to attract enough students of superior ability it may be advisable to draw attention at the earliest opportunity to the limitless career value of nursing in its various branches and to help to raise the level of aspiration of the most adventurous students. People's aims and ambitions appear to be an important aspect of their personality structure. McClelland developed a method of measuring achievement needs of people under various conditions of success and failure. He showed that achievement motive had its origins in childhood. If mothers expected early independence from their sons and showed pleasure in their sons' success by hugging and kissing, they grew up expecting to achieve success later in life. McClelland also drew attention to the link between high achievement motive prevalent in people in some cultural groups and the emphasis on success and achievement in fairy tales and children's stories. Achievement motive has been studied much more extensively in men than in women. It is clear from studies which have already been carried out that achievement motives affect adaptation to work, tolerance of frustration and level of aspiration.

Because nursing is a career with a wide range of scope for people of different personality it seems important to investigate what level of achievement need is desirable for different fields of nursing.

Job satisfaction depends, in large measure, on the opportunities for self-fulfilment. These can arise in social relationships, in the exercise of creative or intellectual effort, in the assumption of responsibility. Recognition and acceptance by others contribute to job satisfaction. Herzberg has shown that dissatisfaction manifests itself in complaints about material things, for example money, poor environment, inferior working conditions. To remove such causes for complaint does not, however, result in improved morale without attention to the need for self-fulfilment.

When morale is not good every aspect of work is affected. Where productivity can be measured reduced output is one indicator of lowered morale. In hospital it was always assumed that the equivalent to productivity could not easily be measured. Revans has shown, however, that for patients suffering from comparable conditions recovery rate is related to the other indications of morale. In the hospital where evidence pointed to high morale patients were discharged more rapidly and even mortality rates were lower than in the hospital where staff morale was poor. Work quality suffers, but again, in nursing it is not easy to observe this. The sensation of fatigue reported by personnel is one sign that work appears to be less enjoyable than formerly. Among the most common results of low morale are: *rapid turnover* in personnel, *absenteeism* and *accident proneness*.

Turnover

There are many good reasons for a person to change his job. In the early years of working life it is common to make several changes before settling down to the chosen career. Once a career has been selected changes in work are usually related to advancement and promotion. Some personal decisions may also indicate making a change. Marriage, or the fact that the family has moved to a new address, may necessitate change. On the whole though, if anyone is happy in his place of work and his choice of career, he does not make too many changes.

If, in any organisation, staff turnover increases very much it is worth while to investigate morale. People who wish to change do not often refer to their dissatisfactions. They tend to find sound reasons why a change has become necessary. It almost appears as if rationalisation is prevalent in such conditions. Investigation of job satisfaction, however, often shows that people who have failed to find congenial friends, who are on bad terms with their fellow workers, who criticise management and leadership are those who leave their work soon after. The people who are most settled are the ones who mention the pleasure they derive from good companionship, who have made close friends among co-workers and who find their superiors at work competent and fair.

It is interesting that people often find the companionship and friendship of their co-workers more important than the relationship with their superiors. If one wishes to raise the morale of an organisation it may be wise to begin by paying attention to friendship patterns in the arrangement of duty rotas.

Absenteeism

People who feel that morale is poor may not actually leave. They may express their dissatisfaction by frequent absenteeism. They often awake in the morning feeling unwell and rather low and they decide to take time off. This is by no means a deliberate and conscious form of malingering. On the con-

trary the people concerned would feel very hurt if it were
suggested that they were ill because they did not look forward
to their day's work.

Genuine illness becomes much more frequent in those who
are unhappy. Feelings of malaise become more troublesome.
When anyone feels psychologically troubled he develops
many organic symptoms which become sufficiently disabling
to warrant staying away from work. When the individual
feels happy in his work conscious of his responsibility and
needed by his fellow workers, he often ignores minor ailments
because work is important. When the worker is not too sure
whether his work is worth while, or when he does not feel
personally wanted, it is easy to give in to minor illness.

Accidents

It may seem surprising that accidents may have psychological significance. By definition an accident appears to be
an event which happens fortuitously with no known antecedents. Yet a study of the circumstances in which accidents
occur often shows that considerable psychological stress
precedes the accident. People who worry suffer from lack of
concentration and so cause accidents. Their anxiety may make
them clumsy and worry may lead to slower reaction time and
therefore accidents are less easily warded off. Loss of sleep and
fatigue may have something to do with accidents. When
people are mentally unwell they may resort to taking drugs
or alcohol which in turn increase the risk of accidents.

When morale is low the accident rate generally rises and
increased damage to property and persons results. Some people
are much more prone than others to have accidents when
they are under stress. In any community a few people between them have most of the accidents while a large number
of people never have accidents at all. People who repeatedly
have accidents are said to be 'accident prone'.

Some psychologists look for a more specific connection between psychological troubles and accident proneness. They feel that certain people behave as if they were punishing themselves by getting hurt. In extreme cases people who are totally oblivious of danger or who enjoy taking risks are people who do not find life worth while. Any sudden increase in accident rate or any serious accident proneness by certain members of staff should lead to investigation of morale.

SUGGESTIONS FOR FURTHER READING

ABEL-SMITH, B. *A History of the Nursing Profession*. London: Heinemann, 1960.

ARGYLE, M. *The Social Psychology of Work*. London: Allen Lane, The Penguin Press, 1972.

BROWN, J. A. C. *Social Psychology of Industry*. Harmondsworth: Penguin, 1954.

GHISELLI, E. E. and BROWN, C. W. *Personnel and Industrial Psychology*. 2nd ed. New York: McGraw-Hill, 1955.

REVANS, R. W. *Standards of Morale: Cause and Effect in Hospital*. London: Oxford University Press (Nuffield Provincial Hospital Trust), 1964.

WARR, P. *Psychology at Work*. Harmondsworth: Penguin, 1971.

25. WORKING WITH OTHER PEOPLE

Very few activities in nursing are carried out in isolation. Most of her working life the nurse works with others or at least in the presence of other people. There is a lot of evidence that behaviour changes in the presence of other people. The term *group dynamics* is used to explain the effect of the group on the individuals who compose it.

A group, in psychological terminology, consists of a number of people who have a common interest, goal or purpose and who form some kind of association with each other because of their common business. If a number of people happen to find themselves at the same place without the bond of common purpose this constitutes a *crowd*. The people travelling in the underground train at the same time, or queuing for tickets for a cricket match, or present at the scene at the time of a road accident have similar interests or aims, but they have not assembled for the purpose of interacting with each other, they form crowds. In a crowd an individual may behave in a markedly different way from his usual standards. Examples have been given of the mass excitement of crowds during political unrest, student demonstrations, at Negro lynchings, anti-Semitic outrages. The individuals concerned would not, singly, have behaved in this way; in fact, often they felt ashamed of their actions. In a crowd they appeared to be less conscious of the controlling influence of their own moral standards and seemed to lose the sense of responsibility for their own actions. Similarly, as one of a crowd, the individual can get more excited and exhilarated by such events as peace celebrations, parades, elections, revivalist meetings. Even the enjoyment of a good concert can be heightened by the presence of an excited audience. Crowd behaviour does not concern us directly when we consider the work of the nurse.

The effect of a group on the functioning of the nurse and on the behaviour of patients is, however, very important. The first group in human life is the family group and we have already shown how experiences in that setting may affect attitudes later in life.

Adults belong to a large number of groups simultaneously and some of these are called *face to face groups*. These groups form when à small number of people meet for the purpose of discussing a problem or carrying out jointly some work project or to enjoy a game, a meal or some conversation. In a face to face group people are affected by the physical presence of others. Face to face groups are sometimes referred to as 'primary groups'.

An individual may belong to many groups without actually meeting their other members. In hospitals the nursing staff forms one group of whom only a few ever meet face to face at any one time. The nursing staff forms a separate group from the medical staff or the domestic staff or the maintenance staff, who have their own groups. The hospital staff as a whole, however, also forms a group with interests and activities concerning all. Nurses may, at the same time, belong to a professional organisation such as the Royal College of Nursing or the Student Nurses' Association. They may also be members of their church, of a political party, perhaps a trade union. These larger groups are referred to as 'secondary' or official groups. In each group different demands may be made upon the nurse; sometimes these are conflicting and create anxiety until the difficulties are resolved.

A sense of belonging appears to be very important to all human beings. More satisfaction may be derived from membership of some groups than from others. In some groups there is a secure feeling of attachment, although a member may sometimes have difficulty in belonging wholeheartedly and may then feel that she is only a 'fringe' member. Sometimes it becomes necessary for a nurse to deal with people to whom she may not feel drawn at all and to whom she may even feel hostile. There may exist a sensation that certain groups of people exclude a would-be member from close membership. Psychologists speak of '*ingroups*' to describe the nucleus of people most closely concerned with membership and of '*outgroups*' to describe those who fail to be integrated into the group or against whom a group appears to operate.

Each group develops its own standards of values, its own rules about behaviour, its own attitudes to which members are expected to conform. When individuals fail to conform the group as a whole exerts pressure to bring the member's behaviour within the range of acceptable behaviour, or else takes action to expel the offender from membership. Groups differ in the degree of variation from the norm that they are able to tolerate and also in the type of sanctions they use against offenders.

Anyone seeking membership in a group is usually attracted by at least part of the group's programme. One person joins a sports club, for example, because he likes its range of sports activities or its facilities, its geographical location, or some of the people in it. Another joins a political party because he agrees with its overall outlook. A third joins a particular hospital because he believes it provides good medical and nursing care. Once a person has become a group member he discovers aspects of which he was not previously aware and which may not be entirely acceptable. The sports club, for example, may have some members whose political opinions the new member does not share; the political party may consist of some individuals whose views on health matters are contrary to what has been expected; the hospital may have developed staff social activities which do not appeal. In order to remain a member of the group the individual must make some compromise and behave in such a way that he does not offend the existing members.

Groups appear to have some kind of independent life of their own. They evolve in an almost predictable manner. During their existence they go through phases of development which are reminiscent of the developmental stages of man. There are early difficulties of group formation and establishment of group norms which resemble childhood and adolescent troubles. They have a period of adult maturity and may finally develop the sluggishness of old age and the degenerative processes of senility. This description refers to the function of the group as a whole, not to the characteristics of any of its individual members. Group standards are formed by the interaction of the members. Once standards are formed individual members are affected by them. Some interesting experiments have thrown light on some details of group interaction.

A classic experiment is that of Sherif. If a small ray of light shines on to a screen in a completely dark room everybody who watches the screen has the impression that the point of light moves. This a universal optical illusion. If people are asked to say how far they think the light has moved they are willing to give an approximate measure. Some people say they saw it move a few inches, others saw it move several feet. When, after individual judgment, people discuss their impressions they change their view and gradually come to an agreement which appears to be a compromise between the different impressions. When the experiment is later repeated each individual's judgment is much nearer the mean than their original estimate. This very simple experiment may appear irrelevant to nursing judgments, but it has served as a standard for other experimental work and it is clear that many judgments are formed by groups of people in the same sort of way. If people are asked to judge the beauty of paintings or the literary value of poetry agreement is reached in a similar way.

Decisions about group actions or about group acceptance or rejection of particular points of view are made by a similar process. Some people in the group appear to have greater influence than others in determining the outcome of discussion. People with great influence are said to have a high prestige in the group. The merits of individual member's remarks are not always examined critically or logically. The higher the prestige of a member the less careful is the examination of his views before they are accepted or incorporated in group decisions. If any particular person's membership is valued by the others he will find his views are more influential than if his continued membership were of no concern to the group. Group attitudes and group standards are therefore much more likely to be changed from within than by any attempt to modify them from outside.

Within a group there can be vigorous argument and violent disagreement without damage to group feeling. The purpose of this is to effect change. If a group is criticised or attacked by an outsider it reacts as a rule by closing its ranks and protecting itself. No modification of views is likely to occur as a result of outside pressure; on the contrary, opinions tend to harden and the group tends to become more rigid in its standards when it is attacked. This process can be seen in action in political parties where vigorous disagreement can occur between people of the same persuasion. The party, however, tends to show a united front to its opponents.

In hospitals where the morale is good there can be very outspoken criticism from within, while all group members have the same purpose of improving existing practices. As soon as an outsider criticises all the staff is united in their defence. In joint consultation staff and management always meet each other after their disagreements have been settled from within and when they can present a unanimous decision to each other.

It has been shown that groups can be more efficient in solving problems than are the individual members. Small groups have been experimentally engaged in solving puzzles or mathematical problems. It was shown that while within a given time no single person solved the problems groups were successful in providing the correct answers. This, of course, happened only when every member of the group concentrated on the problems and was actively trying to co-operate. The hope that committees might be more competent than individuals in solving the complex problems of a hospital is based on the assumption that they are all motivated by the same aim.

When a group is engaged in solving a common problem the more active and also the more silent members are serving a useful function. Often the silent members are the ones who are able to assess all the contributions of the more vocal members. When perhaps in the end the silent member speaks his contribution may be of the utmost importance. During the discussion he may show approval or disapproval, look interested or bored, smile encouragingly or frown in disbelief. The nonverbal participation of a silent group member may make a great deal of difference to the success of a group. In discussion groups or committees it is of interest to see how important are the contributions of each member. Sometimes personal feelings between some of the members may enter into the outcome of the discussion. There may be a tendency for one person always to contradict another or for the group always to accept or veto the suggestions of certain people.

When a decision has been made by a whole group the members feel much more bound by the decision than if it had been imposed on the group by one person. This was shown, for example, when a group of women, after discussion, decided to give some practical help in a volunteer programme to hospitals. When they themselves had made the decision after discussion they acted on it. When they had been persuaded to do so they had said yes, but had done nothing. In making any attempts to help young mothers to change their way of feeding their infants discussion groups are more effective than advice by the health visitor. Decisions about nursing procedures are more likely to be carried out if they are made by the ward sisters themselves.

In every group individual people develop friendships with each other, find that they like some members better than others, benefit more from their association with some, less with others. Individual relationships within the group have an effect on group morale as a whole. The psychologist Moreno has developed a technique of measuring social distance between people which he calls the *'sociometric'* technique. Either by observing people's interaction with each other or by asking questions about it he forms a picture of the choices people make within the group. Someone can be asked who is his best friend; if everyone has one choice only it is soon discovered how often mutual choices occur, how often there are chains of choices: A choosing B, who chooses C, who chooses D. Triangles may form: A choosing B, who chooses C, who chooses A. By allowing more than one choice to each person it is possible to get a clearer picture of the likes and dislikes and particularly to discover who is the most popular in the group and who is isolated. Other observations may show which members of the group are the most active, which the least active, who initiates action, who agrees, and who opposes. Various questions about other people may give an indication of the role each member assumes in the group. Whom do you like best? may reveal the most popular group member. Whose opinion would you ask? might show up the person with most prestige. Who do you think would be most useful in an emergency? might indicate the leader of the group. From the number of mutual choices in the group, the way in which people are connected with others, some valid conclusions can be drawn about the morale of the group.

When group morale is high the group tends to be active and productive. It concerns itself with its main purpose. Group rules are generally accepted and there are few problems of rule enforcement. When a group's morale is low the group as a whole behaves in a very similar way to that in which some neurotically ill people behave. The group resorts to a variety of defence mechanisms which may be successful in keeping it intact but interfere with its productive functioning. In an attempt to increase cohesion between members the group often behaves as if it were attacked by an outside enemy. It feels under attack and reacts by finding a scapegoat. This may be one of the members who is gradually made to leave the group, or more often the group unites in some warfare against another group. Preoccupation with enforcement of rules and preservation of group standards makes it very difficult for change to take place. The normal process of internal argument is suspended and consequently the group becomes resistant to change. Misunderstandings often occur where members of the group are uneasy with each other. This makes the group wide open to rumours. Members of the group believe rumours about each other and about people outside the group and, in turn, contribute to the spread of rumours.

Within the group discussion is often avoided. People feel uneasy with each other. They cannot safely reveal their feelings and consequently hide them and avoid all topics which might arouse strong emotion. The result often is that the group is unable to deal with its business. Instead it chooses neutral topics, resorts to lengthy small talk or explores important topics by indirect reference. This is sometimes seen in meetings in hospital where the most important item on the agenda is never discussed at all or dealt with very briefly while some unimportant point is dealt with at length. Some committees spend an excessive amount of time in discussing food problems. This serves the purpose of testing out the feeling among the members and making it possible to reach agreement on a neutral topic rather than risk disagreement. It is interesting to note how a group settles on some apparently irrelevant topic of discussion and uses it to examine feelings within the group. Someone may, for example, relate the difficulties of a friend of hers in another hospital. The whole group may show great interest and concern and explore at length relationships at that other hospital. All the arguments and anxieties which are relevant to their own group are used, but in reference to the other situation.

Staff Groups in Hospitals

Most of the knowledge about groups is derived either from the therapeutic groups with mentally ill patients or from detailed study of industrial relations. Some applications to hospital are obvious. Recent investigations of staff groups in hospital have proved interesting. The extensive study of morale carried out by Revans and his team in Manchester has shown that the same forces are present in hospital as in industry. Unlike industry, however, the main problems and conflicts among hospital staff are not those of policy or value systems. All are agreed that their collective task is to help the patient as far as they can. The disagreements arise over the way in which each member of the staff evaluates his own and the other members' contributions. Where the ward sisters, for example, feel that the doctors do not pay enough attention to their advice student nurses tend to feel that the ward sisters do not credit them with any ability to contribute. Where the sister feels that the matron would not listen to her or be interested in her problems junior nurses feel the same way about the sister and the patients feel that no one will listen to them.

Among the complaints made by patients those about failure in communications rank very high. The patients' anxiety and uncertainty make it difficult to ask the right question and to find the right person to ask. Nurses, too, are often unable to give the information the patient needs, because they themselves do not know and are too anxious to ask the right question from the right source of information. This process of 'information blockage', created by anxiety and resulting in increased anxiety, tends to pervade the whole hospital structure and can only be remedied when the problem is faced by the entire staff. Anxiety among nurses is frequently very high. Menzies in a study of the defence systems used against anxiety believes that it is in the nature of the situation that nurses bear the full impact of the stress arising from patient care. There are many occasions which arouse strong feelings in the nurse: pity, compassion, love, guilt and fear, disgust and anger, resentment and envy. In addition to the feelings evoked by the patients there are the conflicting feelings in relation to other members of staff, concern with her own status and self-respect, frustrations about learning and teaching, divided loyalties, anxieties about the allocation of priorities where there is more work than can be done and an ever-present sense of personal responsibility often in matters of life and death, even where this responsibility is ultimately not entirely hers. Such permanent acute anxiety is intolerable and defences are essential. Not only does each nurse develop her own defence system, as was shown in an earlier chapter, but the social system of the hospital as a whole serves to reduce anxiety. A system of work-assignments, for example, rather than patient-assignment, shares the responsibility among many and diminishes the intensity of nurse-patient relationships. It allows nurses to treat procedures and symptoms as important rather than people. Adherence to routine reduces the need for decision-making and relieves the individual nurse of the anxiety of responsibility. The hierarchical structure among nursing staff serves an important function in delegating responsibility and removing it from any one person.

While one can understand the traditional nursing structure better if one sees it in relation to the problem of anxiety the recent studies have shown that it does not really work efficiently and that communication difficulties arising from anxiety are central to any attempt to introduce change.

During her training the student nurse may become a member of a small discussion group or of a group working on some educational project. Group work has certain advantages over other forms of instruction, in particular it enables the student to engage in active learning and therefore helps her learn faster and more permanently. One important condition for successful group work, however, is that the student should be willing to learn from her colleagues, respect their views and feel free to offer her own contributions. The psychoanalyst, Bion, has shown that all groups have 'dependency needs', not only therapeutic groups, and that a group can not be effectively task-orientated until its dependency needs have been met. This means that some time in every group, should be devoted to the problems of relationships between members and that efforts should be made to create trust, respect and acceptance.

In recent years methods of monitoring group processes have been developed, in therapeutic groups as well as in administrative and in educational groups. *Bales*, for example, has devised a category system which allows an observer over a period of time to establish which group member is active, positive and constructive and who has the opposite effect on the group. Bales studied verbal and non-verbal contributions. *Flanders* has similarly analysed the behaviour of teachers and students in the classroom.

It is not easy to be, simultaneously, a participant and an observer in a group. Attempts have been made to help people become more sensitive to the dynamics of groups of which they are members. Groups created for the purpose of learning about group dynamics are sometimes referred to as 'T' groups meaning 'training groups'.

SUGGESTIONS FOR FURTHER READING

ARGYLE, M. *The Psychology of Interpersonal Behaviour*. Harmondsworth: Penguin, 1971.

EVANS, K. M. *Sociometry and Education*. London: Routledge & Kegan Paul, 1962.

MENZIES, I. E. P. *The Functioning of Social Systems of Defence against Anxiety*. London: Tavistock, 1961.

MORRISON, A. and MCINTYRE, D. *Social Psychology of Teaching*. Harmondsworth: Penguin, 1972.

26. LEADERSHIP

Whenever a group of people embark on a joint project some form of leadership is required. Even in groups which meet without any specific purpose other than perhaps to play or to converse it soon becomes evident that one person assumes leadership. Sometimes a leader is specifically appointed. Discussion groups, for example, may have a leader appointed for them before the meeting is convened. Football teams or cricket teams have a leader before the team is selected. Appointment to the position of ward sister in hospital or to the nursing officer's job is an appointment to leadership. Officers in the forces are chosen to lead. In industry the foreman, the shop steward, the directors, all have positions of leadership, each of a different kind. The question arises whether certain people have special personality characteristics which give them the ability to lead.

It is well known that some animals adopt a hierarchical order within the herd or flock. Experiments with chickens have shown that the more dominant animals peck the more submissive ones until a definite pecking order emerges. The term 'pecking order' is at times jocularly applied to relationships in human society.

It would appear that leadership qualities do exist in human beings and that suitable education can help people to acquire skills in leadership. To a large extent, however, the characteristics of the group determine the kind of leadership which is required. Every group arranges itself into leaders and followers and adopts the leaders who serve its purpose best. In industry foremen are often chosen because of their superior skill and knowledge of production. The men so chosen have proved their ability to understand the goal of the management and are able to make a substantial personal contribution. It is assumed that their greater skill gives them the necessary prestige and enables them to lead the workers. This often proves to be a fallacy. If the workers were all primarily concerned with the goal of the organisation the foremen so chosen would have greater success. Very frequently, however, the individuals and the various subgroups of individuals have objectives and goals far removed from the overall purpose of the industry. A successful leader takes the changing needs of the small groups into account and aims to make the small groups integrated parts of the entire organisation.

In hospitals, ideally, all employees should be working towards the same goal. However, there are many problems specific to small subsections of personnel. Student nurses have problems of their own not shared by trained staff. Nurses have problems and needs which are special to their work and different from the problems of doctors. Electricians in hospital have special concerns of their own, kitchen staff meet difficulties that other groups fail to notice or understand. Each of these groups and all other subgroups within a hospital require leaders who understand the effect they have on each other. Excellence in nursing or electrical engineering or cooking is not sufficient to make a person acceptable to the group as a leader.

In different situations people may require different leaders. A particular person may satisfy the group while they are all engaged on learning a new technique in their job. His knowledge and teaching skills may render him particularly suitable for leadership. If a fire were to break out an entirely different member of the group might take the initiative to lead people to safety and to avoid panic. If the group decided to form a dramatic society another member would emerge as leader; if they decided to form a cricket team yet another man would be appointed. Where the organisation is sufficiently flexible to allow different people to adopt new roles as the need arises leadership is usually determined by the group itself.

In most situations leaders have to be chosen, trained and appointed although this does not have to preclude the emergence of spontaneous leaders. Ward sisters must be chosen; it cannot be left to the group to select someone to lead a nursing team. A good ward sister makes it possible to allow individual nurses to assume leadership for a special purpose; for example in planning a particular nursing project or in organising the Christmas activities. Good leadership on the part of the Nursing Officer entails discovering the people who can take the initiative in leadership in a large variety of nursing activities. Delegation of responsibility which is part of good leadership is the ability to utilise leadership qualities wherever they are found and to give those who are able to take responsibility the greatest possible scope for independent action and decisions on behalf of their group.

People appointed to leadership can use their position in a variety of ways. These have been described as autocratic, democratic and laissez-faire. The word democratic is not used in a political sense. Broadly speaking autocratic leadership has all authority vested in the leader himself. In democratic leadership responsibility is delegated. In laissez-faire leadership channels of authority and the areas of responsibility are not clearly defined.

An investigation of different types of leadership in youth groups was carried out in America by Lippitt and White and by Lewin. Each group in turn was organised under each of the three forms of leadership. It was found that under laissez-faire leadership there was the smallest amount of constructive or enjoyable activity. Under autocratic leadership the young people functioned well while the leader was there, but all activity ceased when the leader left the room. In the absence of the leader the group became totally disorganised. With democratic leadership the group was most productive, morale was highest and activity continued in the absence of the leader.

Democratic leadership seems to be most desirable to some psychologists, although in some organisations it may be less appropriate. The army, for example, functions well on an autocratic organisation. Many investigations show that industry may do better with democratic leadership and hospitals may be very similar to industry. In small groups democratic leadership often produces the best results though some people feel safer with a more authoritarian approach. Leadership depends for its success on the channels of communication which are available.

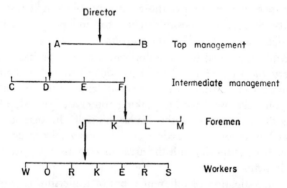

FIG. 11. Downward direction of communication from director to workers.

In some autocratic organisations communication is clearly channelled, but mostly takes place in a downward direction. The directors give instruction to top management. The top management passes it on to intermediate management which in turn passes it on to the foremen who instruct the workers.

There is no official opportunity for people at the same level to discuss with each other or to make their views known to people above them.

In democratic leadership there is a provision for communication between people at each level and for 'feedback'. Each group informs the person who has given the instructions of the outcome of discussions. Difficulties that are anticipated or have occurred as a result of new instructions are discussed and the management is informed of the way in which their plans are received. Upward communication also makes it possible for workers to make suggestions and to take an active part in initiating change.

Some organisations have the necessary machinery for democratic functioning, but it is used in an autocratic manner. There may be meetings of workers, but these are used only for grumbles about unimportant matters. Meetings between workers and management are called but abandoned for want of agenda. Suggestion boxes are available but not used. In such organisations it appears that people in leadership positions are unable to try a democratic organisation. Their reluctance may be due to the fact that a change from autocratic to democratic leadership is often accompanied by a period of relative disorganisation. The belief that democratic leadership in schools is desirable has been gaining ground. In the classroom it can be shown very clearly that the sudden removal of autocratic leadership creates tremendous anxiety. The transition to democratic organisation takes a little time and does not immediately appear to be successful. If a change from autocratic to democratic leadership is to be tried out in industry or in a hospital it may be necessary to prepare for a period of difficulty. It may take a few weeks before meetings and other channels of communication can be used constructively and everybody can be convinced that it is safe to speak.

In small groups the various forms of leadership can be most

clearly observed. Many nurses have had experience of participating at meetings or conferences, for example, where different group leaders have adopted different techniques. Some group leaders act as chairmen in such a way that the members of the group feel free to discuss anything they like. The chairman merely summarises, clarifies or helps the group to return to an important point without too many side issues being pursued. The chairman is interested in the contributions of each member and makes it easier for shy and retiring people to speak. He allows silence to take place while people are thinking or trying to cope with their feelings. Most of the discussion takes place between members of the group. The chairman's remarks are addressed to the group as a whole; the members' remarks are addressed to each other.

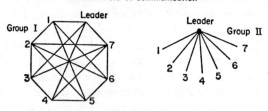

FIG. 12. In Group I members communicate with other members of the group as well as with the leader. In Group II the leader communicates with everyone but the members of the group do not communicate with each other.

Another group leader may take a much more active part. He decides on the choice of the subject, decides what is and what is not relevant. He addresses people individually, calling on them to speak. All remarks are addressed to him.

It is interesting to note the effect of seating on the type of leadership. Some leaders feel that they need a table in front of them or that they like to be seated in a raised position. This clearly marks them off from the group. A barrier is set up between the leader and the group which is symbolic of the relationship he wishes to create for the successful performance of his role. Where the leader wishes to be a member of the group a barrier would be an obstacle to his function. The kind of group in which members communicate with each other is more successful where the room is small, seating informal, preferably in armchairs, where ashtrays are provided and smoking accepted (Group I, Fig. 12).

There are advantages and disadvantages in both types of leadership. Most committee procedure is formal, all remarks addressed to the chair (Group II, Fig. 12). Committees are meant to settle issues efficiently and fairly rapidly after preliminary discussion has already taken place. Preliminary discussion, where all issues should be raised and where it is not yet clear who has the greatest contribution to make, may be more productive in a more informal setting. Hospitals with their large staffs and complex problems may need both types of leadership on different occasions. Both need practice for successful use.

SUGGESTIONS FOR FURTHER READING

ABERCROMBIE, M. L. J. *The Anatomy of Judgement*. Harmondsworth: Penguin, 1969.

BEARD, R. *Teaching and Learning in Higher Education*. Harmondsworth: Penguin, 1970.

BION, W. R. *Experiences in Groups*. New York: Basic Books, 1961. (Soc. Sci. Paperback. London, 1968).

CLEUGH, M. F. *Educating Older People*. London: Tavistock, 1970.

Discussion Method. Bureau of Current Affairs. 2nd ed. London, 1952.

GIBB, C. A. *Leadership*. Harmondsworth: Penguin, 1969.

Group Discussion in Educational, Social and Working Life. Central Council for Health Education. London, 1955.

KLEIN, J. *Working with Groups*, 2nd ed. London: Hutchinson, 1963.

RUESCH, J. and BATESON, G. *Communication*. New York: Norton, 1968.

27. THE PATIENT'S COMMUNITY

The effect patients have on each other has received relatively little attention in general hospitals. In the days when people paid for hospitalisation those who could afford it chose to have single rooms. Only those who had to accept beds in an open ward did so. Even now many patients regret that private rooms are not available to everybody and many people still choose to pay for the amenities of a private room. The convenience of receiving visitors in private and of sleeping in a room alone without disturbance is obvious; but apart from this it is not so certain that it is beneficial for a patient to be alone.

Nurses and doctors often talk and behave as if each patient were being treated as an isolated, separate individual. They ignore the effects of patients on each other, yet these effects may be harmful or most beneficial. Talk about nursing the 'whole patient' refers to the patient's body and mind, his physical and emotional difficulties. The patient's own social background, his family, commitments, his anxieties about wife and children may be remembered, but his new social attachments to patients in the ward may be overlooked.

Patients are often frightened on arrival. Although nurses do everything in their power to reassure the patient there are long periods when he is left alone with his thoughts and with nothing to do but observe other patients. Patients in neighbouring beds are much better able to help than anyone else. If they can confirm that the hospital is good, that nurses are competent and considerate, if they can speak from their own experience the new patient will find comfort much more rapidly than if they increase his fears by tales of terrible happenings. Patients gain confidence by observing the treatment given to other patients quite as much as by their own experience of it. Patients who are ambulant are often able to give assistance or call for help. They are nearly always responsible for the provision of company for one another during the long idle hours of hospital life especially when the most acute phase of the illness is over.

Many patients feel upset about some patients who are in great pain or who are dying. While there is certainly a need to perform many treatments in private in order to spare sensitive patients the distress of watching and being observed very often the knowledge that other patients are worse off is a source of comfort rather than of distress to many patients. Wherever possible arrangements should be made for removing a dying patient to a private room for his own and his relatives' sake. The other patients in the ward are naturally distressed by death, but it has to be faced and it is not necessarily harmful for patients to share in grief. The practice of moving dying patients into a private room may at times cause unnecessary alarm to patients. They may falsely interpret the moving of their own beds as an indication that death is approaching and they may worry about some friend who is being moved for any other reason than his impending death. In a hospital in which all patients were being nursed in the terminal stages of illness Dr C. Saunders found that patients gained strength and courage from comforting each other and from being present to witness the peaceful death of their fellow sufferers.

Patients who are in private rooms and not aware of what is going on elsewhere in the ward may find it much harder to understand the mood of the wards. They may feel neglected when they are kept waiting while nurses are busy, without being able to derive comfort from seeing someone else well nursed. Even in a private room they may feel the depressing effect which death has on the ward and the nurses and they may find it more difficult to deal with their troubled feelings all alone.

It is well known that different wards have entirely different atmospheres. Partly the nursing staff creates the feeling of strain or relaxation, of pessimism or optimism. Partly, however, it is created by the patients themselves. Orthopaedic wards and wards for plastic surgery are sometimes among the most cheerful with the highest morale in spite of the serious condition of some patients. The atmosphere almost certainly helps many patients to accept their disability more readily. Gynaecological wards have an atmosphere quite unlike that found elsewhere. The fact that all patients have important psychological problems in common creates a special kind of bond. The nature of their illness results in a certain amount of secrecy, a characteristic way of joking and talking in a peculiar mixture of lightheartedness and seriousness.

In recent years the atmosphere in children's wards and in geriatric wards has received much attention. The pathetic loneliness of the aged when they are sick in bed is a serious handicap to recovery. Early ambulation and determined attempts not to allow old people to become bedridden have helped to keep patients in touch with each other. In wheelchairs elderly patients are able to sit around a fire, see each other, talk to each other and take an interest in each other. Deafness, shortsightedness and inhibited movement make it too difficult to bridge the conventional distance of beds.

Children's wards have become lively, happy, active places. The effect children have on each other is obvious. Serious problems arise when isolation of a child is absolutely necessary, because a sick child cannot easily overcome loneliness. Widespread use of cubicles without imperative reasons is now no longer practised in children's wards. In playrooms and during school every possible attempt is made to encourage interaction and use it for each child's advantage.

In mental hospitals the therapeutic effect of the community has been recognised much longer, though only recently have systematic attempts been made to study the social aspects of mental hospitals and to make active use of patients' ability to help each other. The atmosphere of the hospital as a whole and of each ward is known to be important. Many patients derive personal benefit from feeling useful to the hospital community. Ward meetings of all kinds are commonly held in mental hospitals. Patients actively participate in discussions, elect their own committee and many take office in patients' organisations. Group psychotherapy offers an opportunity for a special kind of participation in mutual help. A very strong sense of belonging is one of the beneficial factors of this form of therapy. In some mental disorders the patient's own efforts at active participation in therapy are even more important than in others. Psychopathic patients, for example, or alcoholic patients have for so long shown their inability to accept help from others that traditional relationships between nurse or doctor and patient are almost doomed to failure. Where patients begin to feel responsible for their own therapy and become active in helping each other their outlook sometimes changes. They can accept help from each other with less resentment than from staff.

The term 'therapeutic community' was originally coined to describe how, in a particular hospital for psychopathic patients, a community spirit developed which helped many patients to gain self-respect, to cultivate their assets to the fullest degree and to gain control over their antisocial and aggressive tendencies. The need to run such a ward democratically was discussed very fully. It was difficult for the staff to give up their position of superiority and to merge completely with the patient community. In the community the staff had equal rights and obligations, but not superior positions. They constituted the more stable and well-adjusted section of the community, but, with the patients, experienced all the trials and tribulations of communal living and of slowly developing culture patterns.

Not all patients benefit from this extreme form of self-government or need to be included in such a self-directing community. For some patients a more maternal or paternal attitude of staff may be indicated. The benefit of active participation in therapy and in the formation of the hospital community is, however, usually a desirable state of affairs.

Much remains to be done to explore the application of the knowledge gained from social psychology to the treatment of patients and the conduct of hospital affairs.

SUGGESTIONS FOR FURTHER READING

CARTWRIGHT, A. *Human Relations and Hospital Care*. London: Routledge & Kegan Paul, 1964.

JONES, M. *Social Psychiatry in Practice*. Harmondsworth: Penguin, 1968.

EPILOGUE

In the preface to this book it was stated that a knowledge of psychology is necessary for an understanding of the nurse's work. The student who has reached the end of this book will be convinced that a knowledge of nursing is necessary to the understanding of psychology as applied to nursing. It is the same with all basic subjects. They appear difficult until they are applied. Then the interest deepens and everything seems easy and obvious. It is often said that physiology must be learnt before one can study pathology. In reality physiology acquires meaning only when one is confronted with disorders of function. Just so with psychology. Normal, healthy behaviour does not appear worthy of study until one meets examples of emotional disturbance.

Having studied this book early in training it is hoped that the student will feel the urge to read it again as and when practical experience in nursing makes manifest a need for deeper understanding. Not only this book, but some of those mentioned in the text and many others on the library shelves, should be consulted. Appetite for psychology grows with every book one reads. As the reader's nursing experience widens she herself will find examples to illustrate her reading and she will discover the need for more theory to illuminate her practice.

For the expert nurse and the expert psychologist much work remains to be done. As I compiled lists of books for further reading I became aware of the paucity of experimental work carried out in nursing. In the last section of the book it was necessary to take many examples from industry, because too few studies of hospitals have been carried out. Will any reader be inspired to remedy this defect and provide, for inclusion in future editions, new information about psychology in nursing?

INDEX

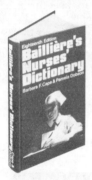
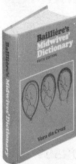
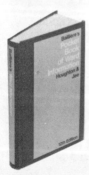

THE NURSES AIDS SERIES ∎⊓⊓⅃⊑

The Nurses' Aids Series is planned to meet the needs of the student nurse during training, and later in qualifying for another part of the Register, by providing a set of textbooks covering most of the subjects included in the general part of the Register and certain specialist subjects. The pupil nurse, too, will find many of these books of particular value and help in practical bedside training. The Series conforms to three factors important to the student:

1. All the authors are nurses who know exactly what the student requires.

ANAESTHETICS FOR NURSES
1971 • 1st edn. • £1.10

ANATOMY AND PHYSIOLOGY FOR NURSES*
1972 • 8th edn. • Limp £1.20 • Hard £2.00

ARITHMETIC IN NURSING
1972 • 4th edn. • Limp £1.10 • Hard £2.00

EAR, NOSE AND THROAT NURSING
1972 • 5th edn. • Limp £1.10 • Hard £2.00

MEDICAL NURSING
1972 • 8th edn. • Limp £1.20 • Hard £2.00

MICROBIOLOGY FOR NURSES*
1972 • 4th edn. • Limp £1.00 • Hard £1.50

OBSTETRIC AND GYNAECOLOGICAL NURSING*
1969 • 1st edn. • Limp £1.20 • Hard £2.00

ORTHOPAEDICS FOR NURSES*
1971 • 4th edn. • Limp £1.20 • Hard £2.00

PAEDIATRIC NURSING
1974 • 4th edn. • Limp £1.30 • Hard £2.00

OPHTHALMOLOGY FOR NURSES
1975 • 1st edn. • Limp £1.20 • Hard £2.00

2. The books are frequently revised to ensure that advances in knowledge reach the student as soon as practicable.

3. The Aids are well printed and easy to read, clearly illustrated, and modestly priced.

Thus this famous Series, which covers all aspects of nursing studies—scientific, theoretical and practical —contributes significantly to nurse training in this country and abroad.

PERSONAL AND COMMUNITY HEALTH
1969 • 2nd edn. • Limp 80p • Hard £2.00

PHARMACOLOGY FOR NURSES
1975 • 4th edn. • Limp £1.20 • Hard £2.00

PRACTICAL NURSING*
1971 • 11th edn. • Limp £1.10 • Hard £2.00

PRACTICAL PROCEDURES FOR NURSES
1969 • 1st edn. • £1.10

PSYCHIATRIC NURSING
1973 • 4th edn. • Limp £1.10 • Hard £2.00

PSYCHOLOGY FOR NURSES
1975 • 4th edn. • Limp £1.20 • Hard £2.00

SURGICAL NURSING*
9th edn. • Limp £1.20 • Hard £2.00

THEATRE TECHNIQUE
1967 • 4th edn. • £1.10

TROPICAL HYGIENE AND NURSING* *New edition in preparation.*

* Available in Educational Low-priced Book Series editions for sale in certain countries only. Leaflet on request.

DO-IT-YOURSELF REVISION FOR NURSES
BOOKS 1, 2, 3, 4, 5 & 6

E. J. HULL and B. J. ISAACS

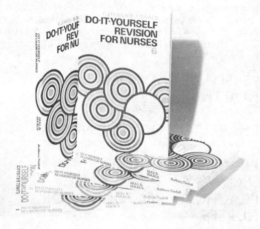

The six books of this series provide a comprehensive framework for revision of the GNC syllabus and developments made since to it. The student reviews a subject of choice, answers questions selected from recent State Final Examinations, and marks her replies against the model answers provided.

'Highly recommended to all student nurses as a planned guide to revision.' *Nursing Times*

'ZRN Finalists and aspiring ZENs would benefit enormously were they to use these little books as intended...Tutors will have cause to be grateful, students even more so.' *Zambia Nurse*

1970-1972 • **Books 1-6** *• 135 pp average • illustrated • Books 1, 2, 3 & 4—70p each • Books 5 & 6—60p each*

BOOKS FOR THE PSYCHIATRIC NURSE

ALTSCHUL/
PSYCHIATRIC NURSING
Indispensable to students training for admission to the Register of Mental Nurses.
1973 • 4th edn. • 400 pp. • Limp £1.10 • Hard £2.00

ACKNER/
HANDBOOK FOR PSYCHIATRIC NURSES
This is the well-known RMPA manual.
1964 • 9th edn. • 364 pp. • 1 illus. • £2.20

BURR/
NURSING THE PSYCHIATRIC PATIENT
For students in psychiatric training.
1970 • 2nd edn. • 303 pp. • 8 illus. • Limp £1.75 • Hard £2.00

PEARCE & MILLER/
CLINICAL ASPECTS OF DEMENTIA
Focuses on the treatable presenile dementias.
1973 • 160 pp. • 12 plates, 15 illus. • £3.00
"Extremely useful,"—Nursing Mirror

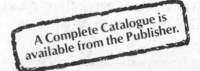
A Complete Catalogue is available from the Publisher.

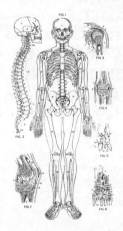